Home Care for Older Adults Using Interprofessional Teams

Danita H. Stapleton • Sekeria Bossie
Editors

Home Care for Older Adults Using Interprofessional Teams

Springer

Editors
Danita H. Stapleton
Department of Rehabilitation Studies, College of Health Sciences
Alabama State University
Montgomery, AL, USA

Sekeria Bossie
Department of Rehabilitation Studies, College of Health Sciences
Alabama State University
Montgomery, AL, USA

ISBN 978-3-031-40891-5 ISBN 978-3-031-40889-2 (eBook)
https://doi.org/10.1007/978-3-031-40889-2

This Springer imprint is published by the registered company Springer Nature Switzerland AG
The registered company address is: Gewerbestrasse 11, 6330 Cham, Switzerland

Paper in this product is recyclable.

To our aging loved ones
May you have the privilege of living in your home and community safely, independently, and comfortably for as long as you desire.
May you be afforded the dignity of aging in place with the support of a skilled interprofessional team who respects your inalienable right to self-determination

Acknowledgments

The completion of this project was made possible by so many wonderful individuals, and we would like to extend our deepest gratitude to you all: To our families, thank you for creating environments that encouraged us to dream big, and for supporting us whenever we chose to chase after those dreams. Thank you for your faith, and for believing that this book could be done and for supporting and encouraging us every step of the way. To our friends and coworkers, thank you for your persistent inspiration and support as we championed this project. To all of the contributing authors, thank you for your hard work, time, and patients as we progressed through this project. We are eternally grateful. We expect that this book will change lives, and we have you all to thank for that. To the Springer Nature publishing team, thank you for your guidance and support throughout the production of this book. A special thank you to Janet Kim and Kausalya Boobalan for granting us the honor to engage in this meaningful work.

Contents

Contributors

Sekeria Bossie, PhD, LPC-S, NCC Department of Rehabilitation Studies, College of Health Sciences, Alabama State University, Montgomery, AL, USA

Scott Bretl, MPO, CPO/L Department of Prosthetics and Orthotics, College of Health Sciences, Alabama State University, Montgomery, AL, USA

Tabitha Brookins, PhD, LMSW Department of Social Work, College of Liberal Arts and Social Sciences, Alabama State University, Montgomery, AL, USA

Ashley Cancer, PT, DPT Department of Physical Therapy, College of Health Sciences, Alabama State University, Montgomery, AL, USA

Dailen Castillo, OTD MBA, OTR Doctor of Occupational Therapy Program, College of Physical Therapy, University of Incarnate Word, San Antonio, TX, USA

Kenya Crews, OTD, MRC, OTR/L Department of Physical Therapy, College of Health Sciences, Alabama State University, Montgomery, AL, USA

Revenda Greene, PT, DPT, PhD Department of Physical Therapy, College of Nursing and Allied Health Sciences, Howard University, Washington, DC, USA

Lenetra Jefferson, PhD, RN, CNE School of Nursing, College of Health and Human Services, Troy University, Troy, AL, USA

Mary-Anne Joseph, PhD, LPC Department of Rehabilitation Studies, College of Health Sciences, Alabama State University, Montgomery, AL, USA

Lovett Lowery, OTD, OTR/L, NBOTC Department of Physical Therapy, College of Health Sciences, Alabama State University, Montgomery, AL, USA

Department of Occupational Therapy, College of Health Sciences, Alabama State University, Montgomery, AL, USA

Jessica Maxwell, PhD, OTD, OTR Doctor of Occupational Therapy Program, School of Physical Therapy, University of the Incarnate Word, San Antonio, TX, USA

Gilaine Nettles, PT, PhD, DPT Department of Physical Therapy, College of Health Sciences, Alabama State University, Montgomery, AL, USA

Letitia Osburn, DHSc, MS, OTR/L Department of Physical Therapy, College of Health Sciences, Alabama State University, Montgomery, AL, USA

Charlene Portee, PT, PhD, FAAPT Department of Physical Therapy, College of Health Sciences, Alabama State University, Montgomery, AL, USA

Tracy Pressley, MS, LICSW Department of Social Work, College of Liberal Arts and Social Sciences, Alabama State University, Montgomery, AL, USA

Jared Rehm, PhD Department of Physical Therapy, College of Health Sciences, Alabama State University, Montgomery, AL, USA

Shanae Shaw, PhD Department of Social Work, College of Liberal Arts and Social Sciences, Alabama State University, Montgomery, AL, USA

Danita H. Stapleton, EdD, LPC-S, CRC Department of Rehabilitation Studies, College of Health Sciences, Alabama State University, Montgomery, AL, USA

Geordan Stapleton, MS, RDN Performance Nutrition Division, New York Mets, Port St. Lucie, FL, USA

Bridgette Stasher-Booker Department of Health Information Management, College of Health Sciences, Alabama State University, Montgomery, AL, USA

Adan Vazquez, M.Ed. CP Department of Prosthetics and Orthotics, College of Health Sciences, Alabama State University, Montgomery, AL, USA

About the Editors

Danita H. Stapleton, EdD, LPC-S, CRC, is the Chairperson of the Department of Rehabilitation Studies at Alabama State University. She has over 30 years of experience in several rehabilitation settings: corrections, forensic rehabilitation, outpatient and in-patient substance use disorder treatment, and intermediate care facilities. Dr. Stapleton has also provided mental health services for older adults in skilled nursing facilities.

Sekeria Bossie, PhD, LPC-S, NCC, is an Assistant Professor at the Department of Rehabilitation Studies, Alabama State University. She has valuable experience working on interprofessional teams composed of varied disciplines. She has provided mental health services for older adults in their natural (home) environment. Dr. Bossie also has experience coordinating and managing home healthcare services for this population.

Chapter 1
Introduction: History of Home Care Services

Sekeria Bossie and Danita H. Stapleton

Learning Objectives

1. Become knowledgeable of legislation and policies relevant to home care service.
2. Become familiar with the risks and benefits of home care services.
3. Be aware of the different types of home care services.
4. Learn about the theoretical perspectives in home care services.
5. Become familiar with care coordination and care models related to home care services.

Introduction

Over the years, nations have witnessed a significant shift in population proportion due to adults living much longer lives. Although some older adults are quite healthy, others have significant or chronic health concerns. Moreover, many experience difficulties adjusting to the physical or mental debility that often accompanies the aging process. The increased longevity of the masses has become a major catalyst for changes in the healthcare field. A notable variation is the increased use of home healthcare services. Although these vital services are offered to diverse groups, older patients have particularly benefited from these services. Home healthcare services are tailored and needs-driven and frequently render positive outcomes. Patients who are older often have complex needs that cannot be met by one single home care provider. Also, receiving care from multiple providers and agencies can be problematic for older patients and their caregivers. Thus, interprofessional collaboration for this population becomes a care necessity.

Supplementary Information The online version contains supplementary material available at https://doi.org/10.1007/978-3-031-40889-2_1.

S. Bossie (✉) · D. H. Stapleton
Department of Rehabilitation Studies, College of Health Sciences, Alabama State University, Montgomery, AL, USA
e-mail: sbossie@alasu.edu; dstapleton@alasu.edu

D. H. Stapleton, S. Bossie (eds.), *Home Care for Older Adults Using Interprofessional Teams*, https://doi.org/10.1007/978-3-031-40889-2_1

The term interprofessional collaboration is used to describe the process by which different health and social care professional groups work together to positively impact the care of a patient [1]. The term *interprofessional* is a relatively new catchphrase signifying healthcare collaborations in general. In recent years, the term has replaced or been interchanged with longstanding terms such as *interdisciplinary* and *multidisciplinary*. Interdisciplinary and multidisciplinary principles of care have significantly advanced patient care and solutions. These expressions should not be devalued. In fact, they serve as the foundation for the more progressive term *interprofessional*. Organizations seeking to bring about successful healthcare change should necessitate that their providers work to accomplish continuative care within integrated interprofessional care systems (ICTs) [2].

There has been emphasis placed on the importance of providers shifting their attention from (organizational or administrative) structures to interpersonal relations and interactions [3]. This is important because healthcare is designed on the principle of boundary drawing with accentuation on role divisions and responsibilities [4]. However, teamwork has proven to be an important aspect in improving patient outcomes and satisfaction. Teamwork has been described as involving two or more care providers with concrete goals surrounding assessment, planning, performing, and evaluating with defining attributes of interdependent collaboration, open communication, and shared decision-making [5]. Additionally, teamwork is defined as an interpersonal process leading to the achievement of goals that cannot be attained by a single member [6]. Five key components of interdisciplinary collaboration have been identified: interdependence, newly created professional activities, flexibility, collective ownership of goals, and reflection on process [6]. Other essential ingredients have been identified as leading to successful interprofessional collaborations [4]. These include respecting the competencies of others, maintaining close interactions, and being flexible and creative. It has been posited that a climate of trust must be continually nurtured for optimal interprofessional collaborations. Additionally, it has been asserted that having no experience and understanding of interprofessional collaborations can hinder members' ability to identify deficiencies while caring for older persons with multimorbidity [3].

Interprofessional collaboration can increase job satisfaction and reduce stress levels [7]. It also affords opportunities for members to resolve stereotypes or preconceptions about other professions. The research literature has emphasized the need for healthcare organizations to not only provide interprofessional education but to afford opportunities for application [7]. Education provides the foundation for building trust among professionals. Additionally, trust must be developed before cooperative processes can be established and implemented. Historical impediments to interprofessional collaboration comprise physician qualities (knowledge, skills, emotions), relational factors (levels of communication and collaboration), and structural factors (organization of care, compartmentalization) [8, 9]. Care deficiencies resulting from a lack of interprofessional collaboration have focused attention on the value of interprofessional teamwork and facilitated initiatives to reduce care gaps [10].

Poor communication and interaction between care team members can adversely influence the knowledge and understanding of patient factors, as well as the quality of community care [11–13]. It has been emphasized that many modern-day medical students are required to participate in interprofessional education [14]. However, for many older rural physicians, such education and awareness opportunities were not available during their medical training. There is a need for all physicians, but particularly those in rural communities, to become proficient in using interprofessional teams effectively. There is also a need for home healthcare professionals to enhance their understanding of care team members' working conditions, roles, and competencies [14]. Such understanding maximizes connectedness and continuity of care, promotes the best possible use of expertise, and reduces unnecessary knowledge gaps. Understanding colleagues' competencies is necessary for effective interprofessional collaboration. If workers from different fields understand each other's skills, then patient information can be shared and practical help can be received [15]. It is emphasized that a prerequisite for interprofessional collaboration is knowledge of other's expertise, roles, and responsibilities [16]. Presently, many healthcare workers perform their tasks independently which results in a lack of sharing of need-to-know information as well as a lack of understanding of care team members' professional abilities.

Patients – especially older adults – with multimorbidity face perils relating to polypharmacy, frequent hospitalization, or high mortality rates when interprofessionalism is lacking [17]. Exchanging information about patients' medical conditions is necessary for smooth multiprofessional cooperation. Problems commonly encountered by home healthcare workers are categorized as biomedical, social, psychiatric, and interprofessional [18]. Interprofessional problems stem from inadequate information sharing, vaguely defined roles, and hierarchy conflict. The shift to team-based care is challenging; however, it is imperative that healthcare providers be equipped with the necessary competencies to work together to accomplish the best possible outcomes for patients who are older [19].

Operating Frameworks: Legislation/Policy and Theoretical Perspectives

Interprofessional collaboration is an ethical and accountable component of healthcare in the home setting. Its function is to guarantee that services are relevant to the needs of patients. Many legislative policies have been established to assure best care practices within the home setting. Table 1.1 presents key legislation from 2013 to 2020. Highlights from each legislative act or policy are included in the table. These have been fundamental in establishing an operating framework for home healthcare. Additionally, there are a few notable home care models and theoretical perspectives that offer an operational framework for home healthcare services. Only a few of these will be discussed in this chapter.

Table 1.1 Legislation/policy

Year(s)	Legislation	Highlights
2013–2014	The Improving Medicare Post-Acute Care Transformation (IMPACT) act of 2014	Required post-acute providers (PAC) to report standardized patient assessment data, data on quality measures, and data on resources and other measures
2016	Twenty-first Century Cures Act of 2016	Required reports on the expanded use of telehealth services and the barriers to such technology in Medicare, new Medicare coverage of home infusion therapy, mandatory use of electronic visit verification in Medicaid home health services
2018	Bipartisan Budget Act of 2018 A. Sec. 50301. Independence at home B. Sec 50323. Increasing convenience for Medicare advantage enrollees through telehealth	A. Extended the Independence at home (IAH) demonstration program for an additional 2 years and 5000 more participants (provided comprehensive primary care in the home, particularly targeted toward beneficiaries suffering from multiple chronic conditions) Starting in 2020, Medicare advantage plans may offer additional telehealth services as supplemental benefits that are available under part B and are identified as clinically appropriate when a medical practitioner is not in the same area as the plan enrollee
2020	Coronavirus Aid, Relief, and Economic Security Act or the CARES act A. Sec. 3707. Encouraging use of telecommunications systems for home health services furnished during emergency periods B. Sec. 3708. Improving care planning for Medicare home health services	A. Directed the Secretary of HHS to consider ways to encourage use of telecommunication systems, including remote patient monitoring, consistent with the plan of care for the individual B. Provided authorization to nurse practitioners, physician assistants, and clinical nurse specialists to certify Medicare beneficiaries' eligibility for home health services
2021	American Rescue Plan Act A. Sec. 9817. Additional support for Medicaid home care- and community-based services during the COVID-19 emergency	Provided for a 10% increase for 1 year starting on April 1, 2021, to the Federal Medical Assistance Program, the federal share of Medicaid, specifically, for home care-based services. These funds can be applied toward home health care services, personal care services, PACE services, HCBS services, case management services, and rehabilitation services
2021	CONNECT for Health Act of 2021	Promotes higher quality of care, increased access to care, and reduced spending in Medicare through the expansion of telehealth services
2021	Choose Home Care Act of 2021	A cost-effective and patient preferred home-based extended care benefit supplemental to the existing home health benefit that supports patients to leave the hospital and recover at home with a mix of expanded skilled nursing therapy, personal care, telehealth services, and more

Theoretical Care Perspectives (Specific to Understanding Patients' Perspective)

Systems Theory

This theory describes human behavior in terms of complex systems [20]. It considers the person in relation to multiple systems. This theory considers how the systems work together. This theory is designed on the structures and subsystems that surround a service user [20]. This theory also recognizes that any change in one part of the system tends to have repercussions for other parts of the system [20]. Understanding this ripple effect is vital when providing in-home care to older patients. Additionally, systems theory is premised on the idea that an effective system considers the patient's needs, rewards, expectations, and the attributes of others living in the system [20]. Older patients may have many people in their systems. Understanding those individuals' needs, rewards, expectations, and attributes is just as important as understanding those concepts for the patient. According to this theory, families and agency members have the capacity to directly resolve problems.

Biopsychosocial-Spiritual Approach

This approach assesses the various levels of functioning within the biological, psychological, social, and spiritual dimensions and helps to explain how they are connected to understanding human behavior. Examining each of the dimensions below will promote more holistic exploration and assessment of the patient who is older [20].

Biological : comprises overall health, physical abilities, weight, diet, lifestyle, medication/substance use, gender, and genetic connections/vulnerabilities.

Psychological : comprises mental health, self-esteem, attitudes, beliefs, temperament, coping skills, emotions, learning, memory, perceptions, and personality.

Social : comprises peer and family relationships, social supports, cultural traditions, education, employment, socioeconomic status, and societal messages.

Spiritual : comprises aspects related to spiritual or religious beliefs or being supported or feeling connected to a higher power or being.

Ecological Theory

The ecological theory of aging suggests that the environment influences the elder's functional status, and the interaction between the individual and the environment is continuously changing. Promoting optimal outcomes requires the goodness of fit between the patient and the environment [21]. For example, the person-environment fit can positively or negatively influence health outcomes if personal competencies are well-suited or poorly matched to environmental demands. The World Health Organization (WHO) Report on Ageing and Health highlights the importance of environmental influences on functioning. The older patient's opportunities to build and maintain functional abilities are enhanced when living in an environment that addresses personal needs [22].

Theoretical Perspectives (Specific to Rehabilitation Theory Models)

There have been many opinions and models that have cultivated the home care field. Three pioneer theoretical perspectives specific to home care services are described in Table 1.2. These perspectives expand over a period of several decades and offer a lens for viewing and understanding the practices and principles that guide the delivery of home care. Commonalities between the three models comprise the following concepts: person-centeredness, biopsychosocial influences, self-sufficiency, autonomy, and interrelationships.

Overall, rehabilitation theory models have evolved around the concept of self-care management. When self-care independence is not possible, the patient is assisted to do as much as possible without pain, loss of quality of life, or the progression of disability [23]. Central to rehabilitation theory models is the provision of home services that assist the patient, encourage adaptation, and channel the resources that are needed [23].

When providing services to patients who are older, it is vitally important that home healthcare providers function synchronously toward common goals. Very often these patients have multiple caregivers and multiple professionals addressing different ailments or conditions. Maneuvering through these complex circumstances requires a high level of communication, teamwork, knowledge, and various other factors that promote active and purposeful interprofessional collaboration.

IPEC Model of Care

Interprofessionalism fosters a care delivery context wherein healthcare professionals can cooperatively exchange knowledge for the betterment of their home care patients. Interprofessional practices facilitate shifts from fragmented services to well-informed collaborative interventions. Additionally, interprofessional teams "develop unified plans for patient assessment and treatment, and all members are considered to be colleagues who have a range of both unique and overlapping skills that contribute to patient care and team functioning" [26]. Within this concept, team members share responsibility for the effective functioning of the team and share

Table 1.2 Rehabilitation theory models

Theoretical model	Influencer	Description
The Albrecht Model for Home Health Care of 1990	Mary Nies Albrecht	This model emphasized patient self-care with emphasis on the following concepts: Accessibility, availability, continuity, cost-effectiveness, demand, intervention, client classification, accountability, comprehensiveness, coordination, efficiency,productivity, quality of care, and use of theme care [23]. This model champions an in-depth focus on the consumers and the many factors guiding and impacting the provision of services. Intrinsic to the model are the assumptions that clients and families are capable of making independent decisions about the setting of care goals [24]. This model reflects the complex nature of home healthcare and the relationship dynamics among the structure, process, and outcomes and is based on the interrelationships among all those involved [24]
Self-Care Deficit Nursing Theory (1959–2001)	Dorothea Orem	The central philosophy is that all patients want to care for themselves (autonomy). It is believed that patients with greater autonomy are able to recover more quickly and holistically by performing their own self-care as much as they are able to. The general concepts of Orem's theory consist of self-care, self-care agency, therapeutic self-care demand, and self-care requisites [25]. There are three self-care requisites: Universal self-care, developmental self-care, and health deviation [25]. These requisites consist of a multitude of activities that are essential to everyday living. This model asserts that when there is an insufficiency in either of these three requisites, there will be a deficit in care [25]. Using this model when a deficiency exists, professionals provide a service or intervention that aids the patient in being able to function as independently as possible in their natural environment
The Rice Model of Dynamic Determination 1996	Robyn Rice	This framework is patient-focused and incorporates the patient's perceptions, motivations, health beliefs, sociocultural influences, support systems, and disease process [23]. In this model the nurse, patient, and caregiver move through stages of dependence, interdependence, and independence together to achieve as much independence as possible in the home [23]. The ultimate goal is for the patient to be able to manage their healthcare needs in order to achieve personal harmony [23]

leadership functions" [26]. The Interprofessional Education Collaborative (IPEC) introduced four core competencies for promoting collaborative care. Those who embrace the principles of interprofessionalism:

> (a) work with individuals of other professions to maintain a climate of mutual respect and shared values; (b) use knowledge of one's own role and those of other professions to appropriately assess and address healthcare needs of patients and to promote and advance the health of the population; (c) communicate with patients, families, communities, and professionals in health and other fields in a responsive and responsible manner that supports a team approach to the promotion and maintenance of health and the prevention and treatment of disease; and (d) apply relationship-building values and the principles of team dynamics to perform effectively in different team role to plan, deliver, and evaluate patient-centered care and population health programs and policies that are safe and timely. [26]

Overall, the IPEC Model of Care exemplifies an atmosphere of respect, professionalism, collaboration, and high performance. The model promotes seamless care delivery and promotes both physical and psychological safety for patients and families. Under this care model, there are fewer errors in assessment and decision-making and reduced risk of service duplication.

Benefits of Home Healthcare Services

For the patient who is older, the home care milieu illuminates alternative and holistic perspectives that are not always discernible in an office or hospital setting. Home care is particularly beneficial for persons who are older who are certified as homebound. For homebound individuals, leaving home for medical treatment is often not a viable or convenient option [27]. Older patients demonstrating cognitive impairment and mobility limitations are ideal candidates for home care services. In general, an older patient is a candidate for home services if leaving the home poses a medical risk or is contraindicated [28].

Benefits of interprofessional teaming such as patient satisfaction, seamless care coordination, and improved health outcomes have long been acknowledged. However, when these collaborations occur within the home milieu, other patient benefits are evident: (a) decreased hospital readmissions, (b) improved daily functioning, (c) reductions in health costs, (d) better informed decision-making by providers, and (d) more accurate patient assessments [29]. Other advantages of home care include reduced exposure to infectious diseases, as well as significant cost savings to the Medicare program when compared to skilled nursing facility costs [30]. The provision of home healthcare services can create stronger provider-patient relationships, enhance understanding of patients' environment and support systems, reduce or eliminate travel to and from medical facilities, and lessen stress levels for patients and their families [28].

Types of Home Healthcare Services

Overall, home health services are diverse. A typical service listing comprises physician care, skilled nursing, medical social work, physical therapy, speech therapy, occupational therapy, homemaking, and personal assistant care. Other services may include durable medical services, prosthetics and orthotics services, pharmacy services, and nutritional services. In the ensuing chapters, the readers will learn more about specific home healthcare providers, their roles on the interprofessional team, and their unique perspectives and functions. Home care services are typically authorized by a physician or allowed practitioner and in accordance with a care or treatment plan.

Care Coordination Between Interprofessional Team Members

Well-coordinated, integrated home care services allow older persons with diverse health conditions to maintain their health, quality of life, dignity, and independence as long as possible. Extant research findings point to inadequate collaborations between physicians and other medical professionals. This lack of effective communication between physicians and other medical professionals can lead to a high patient mortality rate in hospitals and home care settings [31, 32].

The United Nations projected that a person aged 65 in 2015–2020 could expect to live, on average, an additional 17 years [33]. It is expected that, by 2045–2050, figure will increase to 19 years [34]. As the population ages, many individuals will require more (yet different types of) supportive medical services to help them manage medications, perform necessary activities of daily living, and enjoy the highest quality of life possible [35]. Given the growing number of older individuals with chronic diseases, there is a push to decrease the number of inpatient admissions and to increase the percentage of in-home rehabilitation. Rehabilitation or recuperation initiatives in the home setting promote improved patient outcomes because care interventions are better aligned with activities of daily living and local services and resources. Home-based care has proven to be effective for survivors of strokes, patients with dementia, and patients with musculoskeletal conditions, where coordinated services among interprofessional teams are necessary [36–41].

Research has emphasized the value of multicomponent restorative home-based services [42]. Some advantages included improvements in morale, self-care and mobility, activities of daily living, and home management. Overall, multicomponent restorative home-based services resulted in a reduced need for extended services [42]. Additionally, it has been surmised that multicomponent restorative services must be timely and educational and include assistive technologies to encourage patients to continue independence and former activities [42]. Multicomponent restorative home-based services "align more closely with recent models of healthy aging and the progressive principles of service provision already well-established among other disabled groups, with their emphasis on independence, empowerment and community-based treatment" [42].

As late as the 1960s, 40% of medical consultations were being done at home, but by the 1980s, this number had declined significantly to less than 1% [43]. The reasons for the decline in medical home visits were due to factors such as the development of more convenient transportation systems, limited resources available within the home setting or within the physician's large Gladstone (doctor's) bag, and the rapid increase in specializations among physicians. The increase in specializations reduced the number of general practitioners (GPs) who tended to be more skilled at handling diverse health concerns [42].

Interprofessional care teams (IPCTs) are the basis for real collaboration, promoting an environment that is complete, inclusive, and holistic for patients who are older ([44, 45]). Additionally, IPCTs' commitment to cohesion and constant dialog fosters better care planning [46, 47]. These efforts allow for transparent communication among the professionals so that each professional on the interprofessional care team is aware of the intentions and exertions of the other.

Some healthcare providers for older patients demonstrated positive intention to engage in interprofessionalism and shared decision-making (IP-SDM) [47]. However, there was a distinct "behavior-intent" gap due to cognitive attitude, affective attitude, time constraints, perceived behavioral control, and lack of human resources. Of the aforementioned, the time factor (having enough time) was frequently an impediment to interprofessional collaboration [48]. Moreover, collaborative work is often intensive and not billable or reimbursable. This means that interprofessional collaboration, while directly beneficial to patients, pulls professionals away from the provision of services that they can be compensated for. This further means that healthcare administrators who desire to implement interprofessional principles must develop clear policies that outline and support the inner workings of interprofessionalism. Many have stressed the importance of developing organizational policies that consider measures for evaluating and sustaining interprofessional team activities [48]. The value of interprofessional education and interprofessional teamwork is described in the passage below [45]:

> Interprofessional education is a social learning activity in which health practitioners in different professions learn with, from, and about each other. Lack of respect for other health professions and stereotypical views can interfere with teamwork and collaboration. Effective teamwork takes work, a fact not explicitly recognized in health care. Medical education has traditionally not taught teamwork and interprofessional communication skills. Opportunities need to be created for health professionals to learn together.

Quality Measures for Home Health Care

Assessing the quality of services provided by interprofessional teams is significantly important. There are a multitude of quality measures that can be used to evaluate home healthcare services from initiation to termination [49, 50]. Typically, when discussing quality measures in healthcare systems, three core areas are highlighted in the research literature. See Table 1.3. Noteworthy is that CMS also champions these quality measures. Outcome measures, process measures, and patient-reported outcomes are fundamental in determining the divide between home care service delivery and patient and family expectations. Quality measures should equate with performance measures. Acceptable quality measures are quantifiable and lead to both patient and system improvements.

In addition to the core areas presented above, two other quality components are frequently discussed in the literature: structure (described as the capacity of the professional to respond to patient needs) and patient features (described as clinical demographics and preference factors that impact treatment options). When it comes to continuous quality (care) improvements, it is imperative that frequent and transparent discussions occur. Every member of the team is responsible for the

Table 1.3 Measures used to assess the quality of home healthcare services

Type of measures	Examples
Outcome measures	Improvement measures
	Measures of potentially avoidable events
	Utilization of care measures
	Cost/resource measures
Process measures	Timely initiation of care
	% of patients with an admission and discharge functional assessment and a care plan that address function
	Drug education on all medications provided to patient/caregiver during all episodes of care
	Influenza immunization received, offered, and refused for current flu season
	Influenza immunization contraindicated
	Drug regimen review conducted with follow-up
Patient-reported outcomes	A patient-reported outcome is a health outcome directly reported by the patient who experienced it

implementation of quality services. Hence, members must do their due diligence and hold fellow members accountable for the lack thereof.

Chapter Summary

This book provides a collective learning forum that generates opportunities for various professions to learn about each other and develop the needed respect and good will that will be mutually beneficial to all (e.g., patients, families, providers). This book accentuates salient characteristics of interprofessional team members and how interprofessional collaboration can benefit patients who are older and desirous of rehabilitating, recovering, and aging in place. The population of individuals over the age of 65 is growing globally. Healthcare professionals' reluctance to collaborate interprofessionally places this high-risk population at even greater risk. Interprofessional collaboration requires stepping outside of professional silos and engaging in meaningful discussions about patient care and team members' expertise, work tasks, and challenges. It is the authors' hope that this book will serve as a basis for improved communication and teamwork among interprofessional team members, particularly those serving patients who are older.

Discussion Question

1. Explain the significance of quality measures and measures of quality assurance in healthcare systems

Multiple Choice Questions

1. What legislation aided patients in leaving the hospital to recover at home with a mix of expanded services such as skilled nursing therapy, personal care, telehealth services, and more?
   (a) Choose Home Care Act
   (b) CONNECT for Health Act
   (c) Affordable Care Act
   (d) Century Cures Act
2. What individuals are most appropriate for home healthcare services?
   (a) Those with low IQs
   (b) Those with mobility limitations
   (c) Those with severe medical conditions
   (d) B and C
3. Which of the following is a benefit of home healthcare services?
   (a) Reduced exposure to infectious diseases
   (b) Provision of informal medical care
   (c) Significant cost savings to the Medicare program
   (d) A and C
4. Which of the following is not considered a home healthcare service?
   (a) Companion care
   (b) Occupational therapy
   (c) Skilled nursing
   (d) Physical therapy
5. What is the fundamental purpose of this book?
   (a) To identify providers who play significant roles in the provision of home healthcare services to patients who are older
   (b) To promote understanding of the care needs of older patients
   (c) To foster collaborative relationships among home healthcare professionals who provide care to older patients in the home setting
   (d) To provide definitions of interprofessional collaboration

References

1. Reeves, S., Pelone, F., Harrison, R., Goldman, J., & Zwarenstein, M. (2017). Interprofessional collaboration to improve professional practice and health outcomes. *Cochrane Database of Systematic Reviews, 6*, CD000072.
2. Salerno, D. (2014). Change management in healthcare public services: Home care models with e-health for the elderly or frail patients with chronic diseases. *International Journal of Integrated Care, 14*(6). https://doi.org/10.5334/ijic.1613

3. Larsen, A., Broberger, E., & Petersson, P. (2017). Complex caring needs without simple solutions: The experience of interprofessional collaboration among staff caring for older persons with multimorbidity at home care settings. *Scandinavian Journal of Caring Sciences, 31*(2), 342–350. https://doi.org/10.1111/scs.2017.31.issue-2
4. Vangen, S., & Huxham, C. (2005). Nurturing collaborative relations. *Journal of Applied Behavior Science, 39*(1), 5–31.
5. Sims, S., Hewitt, G., & Harris, R. (2015). Evidence of collaboration, pooling of resources, learning and role blurring in interprofessional healthcare teams: A realist synthesis. *Journal of Interprofessional Care, 29*(1), 20–25.
6. Bronstein, L. R. (2003). A model for interdisciplinary collaboration. *Social Work, 48*(3), 297–306.
7. Toth-Pal, E., Fridén, C., Asenjo, S. T., & Olsson, C. B. (2020). Home visits as an interprofessional learning activity for students in primary healthcare. *Primary Health Care Research & Development, 10*(21), e59. https://doi.org/10.1017/S1463423620000572
8. Mitchell, G. K. (2002). How well do general practitioners deliver palliative care? A systematic review. *Palliative Medicine, 16*(6), 457–464.
9. Pype, P., Stess, A., Wens, J., Van den Eynden, B., & Deveugele, M. (2012). The landscape of postgraduate education in palliative care for general practitioners: Results of a nationwide survey in Flanders Belgium. *Patient Education and Counseling, 86*(2), 220–225.
10. Yuen, K., Behrndt, M., Jacklyn, C., & Mitchell, G. (2003). Palliative care at home: General practitioners working with palliative care teams. *Medical Journal of Australia, 179*(6), S38–S40.
11. Chen, C. C., & Chiu, S. F. (2009). The mediating role of job involvement in the relationship between job characteristics and organizational citizenship behavior. *The Journal of Social Psychology, 149*(4), 474–494.
12. Matziou, V., Vlahioti, E., Perdikaris, P., Matziou, T., Megapanou, E., & Petsios, K. (2014). Physician and nursing perceptions concerning interprofessional communication and collaboration. *Journal of Interprofessional Care, 28*(6), 526–533.
13. Franklin, C. M., Bernhardt, J. M., Lopez, R. P., Long-Middleton, E. R., & Davis, S. (2015). Interprofessional teamwork and collaboration between community health workers and healthcare teams: An integrative review. *Health Services Research and Managerial Epidemiology, 2*. https://doi.org/10.1177/2333392815573312
14. Ohta, R., Yoshinori, R., Sato, M., Maeno, T., Bond, J., Jagger, C., et al. (2020). Challenges of using ICT regarding acute conditions in rural home care: A thematic analysis. *Journal of Interprofessional Education & Practice, 20*(100349). https://doi.org/10.1016/j.xjep.2020.100349
15. Hallin, K., Kiessling, A., Waldner, A., & Henriksson, P. (2009). Active interprofessional education in a patient-based setting increases perceived collaborative and professional competence. *Medical Teacher, 31*(2), 151–157.
16. Légaré, F., Stacey, D., Pouliot, S., Gauvin, F. P., Desroches, S., Kryworuchko, J., et al. (2011). Interprofessionalism and shared decision-making in primary care: A stepwise approach towards a new model. *Journal of Interprofessional Care, 25*(1), 18–25.
17. Chi, W. C., Wolff, J., Greer, R., & Dy, S. (2017). Multimorbidity and decision-making preferences among older adults. *The Annals of Family Medicine, 15*(6), 546–551.
18. Morris, D., & Matthews, J. (2014). Communication, respect, and leadership: Interprofessional collaboration in hospitals of rural Ontario. *Canadian Journal of Dietetic Practice and Research, 75*(4), 173–179.
19. Kao, H., Conant, R., Soriano, T., & McCormick, W. (2009). The past, present, and future of house calls. *Clinics in Geriatric Medicine, 25*(1), 19–34.
20. Taylor, S. (2020). *Human behavior and the social environment I*. University of Arkansas Libraries.
21. Lawton, M., & Nahemow, L. (1973). *Ecology and the aging process* (pp. 619–674). American Psychological Association.

22. Beard, J., Officer, A., & Cassels, M. (2016). The world report on aging and health. *The Gerontological Society of America., 56*(S2), S163–S166.
23. Neal-Boylan, L. (2011). Theoretical frameworks that support home care. *Clinical Case Studies in Home Health Care., 1*, 5–12.
24. Albrecht, M. (1990). The Albrecht nursing model for home health care: Implication for research, practice, and education. *Public Health Nursing., 7*(2), 118–126.
25. Naz, S. (2017). Application of Dorothea Orem's theory into nursing practice. *Journal of Rehman Medical Institute, 3*(3–4), 46–50.
26. IPEC. *Interprofessional Education Collaborative: Core Competencies for interprofessional practice: 2016 Update*. Retrieved from https://ipec.memberclicks.net/assets/2016-Update.pdf
27. Centers for Medicare and Medicaid. (2020). *Medicare home health benefit* (pp. 1–9). United States Department of Health and Human Services.
28. Mitzner, T. L., Beer, J. M., McBride, S. E., Rogers, W. A., & Fisk, A. D. (2009). Older Adults' needs for home health care and the potential for human factors interventions. *Proceedings of the Human Factors and Ergonomics Society Annual Meetin, 53*(1), 718–722. https://doi.org/10.1177/154193120905301118
29. Stapleton, D. H. (2021). Interprofessional collaborations: Delivering quality home care services to patients who are elderly. *Journal of Rehabilitation Practices and Research, 2*(2), 128. https://doi.org/10.33790/jrpr1100128
30. National Association for Home Health Care and Hospice. (2022).
31. Schweizer, A., Morin, D., Henry, V., Bize, R., & Peytremann-Bridevaux, I. (2017). Interprofessional collaboration and diabetes care in Switzerland: A mixed-methods study. *Journal of Interproffesional Care, 31*(3), 351–359.
32. Tang, C. J., Zhou, W. T., Chan, S. W., & Liaw, S. Y. (2018). Interprofessional collaboration between junior doctors and nurses in the general ward setting: A qualitative exploratory study. *Journal of Nursing Management, 26*(1), 11–18.
33. United Nations, Department of Economics and Social Affairs Population Division World. (2019). *Population Ageing 2019: Highlights*. Retrieved from https://www.un.org/en/development/desa/population/publications/pdf/ageing/WorldPopulationAgeing2019-Report.pdf
34. United Nations. World Population Ageing 2019. Department of Economic and Social Affairs Population Division 2019.
35. Lanoix, M. (2017). No longer home alone? Home care and the Canada health act. *Health Care Analysis, 25*(2), 168.
36. Lincoln, N. B., Walker, M. F., Dixon, A., & Knights, P. (2004). Evaluation of a multiprofessional community stroke team: A randomized controlled trial. *Clinical Rehabilitation, 18*(1), 40–47.
37. Wade, D. T. (2005). Describing rehabilitation interventions. *Clinical Rehabilitation, 19*(8), 811–818.
38. Graff, M. J., Vernooij-Dassen, M. J., Thijssen, M., Dekker, J., Hoefnagels, W. H., & Rikkert, M. G. (2006). Community based occupational therapy for patients with dementia and their caregivers: Randomised controlled trial. *BMJ, 333*(7580), 1196. https://doi.org/10.1136/bmj.39001.688843
39. Dawes, H., Korpershoek, N., Freebody, J., Elsworth, C., Van Tintelen, N., Wade, D. T., et al. (2006). A pilot randomised controlled trial of a home-based exercise programme aimed at improving endurance and function in adults with neuromuscular disorders. *Journal of Neurology, Neurosurgery & Psychiatry, 77*(8), 959–962.
40. Fisher, R. J., Gaynor, C., Kerr, M., Langhorne, P., Anderson, C., Bautz-Holter, E., et al. (2011). A consensus on stroke: Early supported discharge. *Stroke, 42*(5), 1392–1397.
41. Stolee, P., Lim, S. N., Wilson, L., & Glenny, C. (2012). Inpatient versus home-based rehabilitation for older adults with musculoskeletal disorders: A systematic review. *Clinical Rehabilitation, 26*(5), 387–402.
42. Ryburn, B., Wells, Y., & Foreman, P. (2009). Enabling independence: Restorative approaches to home care provision for frail older adults. *Health and Social Care in the Community, 17*(3), 225–234.

43. Bowman, M. A., Lucan, S. C., Rosenthal, T. C., Mainous, A. G., 3rd, & James, P. A. (2017). Family medicine research in the United States from the late 1960s into the future. *Family Medicine, 49*(4), 289–295.
44. Behm, J., & Gray, N. (2012). Interdisciplinary rehabilitation team. In *Rehabilitation nursing: A contemporary approach to practice* (pp. 51–62).
45. Sargeant, J., Loney, E., & Murphy, G. (2008). Effective interprofessional teams: "contact is not enough" to build a team. *The Journal of Continuing Education in the Health Professions, 28*(4), 228–234. https://doi.org/10.1002/chp.189
46. Gougeon, L., Johnson, J., & Morse, H. (2017). Interprofessional collaboration in health care teams for the maintenance of community-dwelling seniors' health and Well-being in Canada: A systematic review of trials. *Journal of Interprofessional Education & Practice, 7*, 29–37.
47. Légaré, F., Stacey, D., Brière, N., Fraser, K., Desroches, S., Dumont, S., et al. (2013). Healthcare providers' intentions to engage in an interprofessional approach to shared decision-making in home care programs: A mixed methods study. *Journal of Interprofessional Care, 27*(1), 214–222. https://doi.org/10.3109/13561820.2013.763777
48. Steffen, A. M., Zeiss, A. M., & Karel, M. J. (2014). Interprofessional geriatric healthcare: Competencies and resources for teamwork. In N. Parchana & K. Laidlaw (Eds.), *Oxford handbook of clinical Geropsychology* (pp. 732–749). Oxford University Press.
49. Donabedian, A. (1985). The epidemiology of quality. *Inquiry, 22*(3), 282–292.
50. Shaughnessy, P. W., & Kurowski, B. (1982). Quality assurance through reimbursement. *Health Services Research, 17*(2), 157–183.

Chapter 2
Professionalism and Ethical Considerations

Lovett Lowery and Charlene Portee

Learning Objectives

1. Define and discuss the importance of professionalism throughout the provision of home care services.
2. Discuss various concepts related to ethics and ethical behaviors.
3. Explore and discuss three professional dispositions required by the home care professional.
4. Identify three aspects of professional conduct.
5. Discuss procedures for maintaining HIPAA compliance and confidentiality while providing home care services.
6. State the purpose of clinical documentation, describe its key elements, and explain how it impacts reimbursement.
7. Describe the common types of older adult abuse, and outline risk factors.
8. Identify signs of common types of adult maltreatment.
9. Describe the reporting requirements for suspected maltreatment, and summarize strategies to prevent it.
10. Define cross-cultural communication and cross-cultural differences, and describe the concepts/conceptual frameworks of different cross-cultural communication models and their implications.
11. Recognize cultural barriers to cross-cultural communication and how cultural biases impact them.

Supplementary Information The online version contains supplementary material available at https://doi.org/10.1007/978-3-031-40889-2_2.

L. Lowery (✉)
Department of Physical Therapy, College of Health Sciences, Alabama State University, Montgomery, AL, USA

Department of Occupational Therapy, College of Health Sciences, Alabama State University, Montgomery, AL, USA
e-mail: llowery@alasu.edu

C. Portee
Department of Physical Therapy, College of Health Sciences, Alabama State University, Montgomery, AL, USA
e-mail: cportee@alasu.edu

D. H. Stapleton, S. Bossie (eds.), *Home Care for Older Adults Using Interprofessional Teams*, https://doi.org/10.1007/978-3-031-40889-2_2

12. Analyze and discuss examples of positive and negative consequences for effective and ineffective cross-cultural communication and basic skills for developing effective cross-cultural communication.

Professionalism in Home Care

Over recent years, the life expectancy for the aging adult in both the present and future societies has been greatly extended, thereby increasing our older adult population. According to the Social Security Administration, "about one out of every four 65-year-olds will live past age 90, and one out of ten will live past age 95" [1]. Older adults often suffer from multiple health conditions and seek health-related services from various healthcare providers in different settings [2, 3]. Some of these settings include hospitals, rehabilitation centers, outpatient clinics, skilled nursing facilities, and the client's home. To ensure the success of the aging process, the healthcare society will be faced with the critical responsibility of promoting and maintaining the health and well-being of this aging population along the continuum of care settings [3]. However, this will not be the only challenge healthcare providers will encounter. With the demographic changes of the older population, the COVID-19 pandemic, and the growing number of health-related services being provided to older individuals in the home care setting [4], it is important that the provision of quality services for this population be extended beyond the healthcare facility and into the home setting. When considering the various interprofessional services provided in the home, such as social work, nursing, physical therapy, occupational therapy, behavioral health, and others, many may focus more on the specific services provided by each individual discipline and less on concepts pertaining to professionalism and ethics. While the professional expectations and ethical guidelines vary across each discipline, these concepts are the cornerstone to quality and efficient service delivery.

Professionalism Defined

Professionalism is a term that most people are familiar with. Most individuals expect professionalism when they are receiving services in structured environments such as facilities and medical offices. With the provision of services in the home, understanding how to provide quality, personable yet professional services is important. "Due to the increasing need and demand of the community for professional healthcare personnel in the home and improving the quality of services, professionalism and acts of professionalism have become key issues in health care systems" [4]. To fully understand the importance of professionalism throughout the provision of home care services, one must know what professionalism is. Professionalism is defined as "the conduct, aims, or qualities that characterize or mark a profession or a professional" [5], and it consists of one's professional parameters, behaviors, and responsibilities [6]. Although this interpretation may appear simplistic in meaning, professionalism has been defined by some as a multifaceted and multidimensional approach, framework, and process, as well as a phenomenon that is both formally and informally taught [4, 6, 7]. Professionalism encompasses several basic, yet important, dispositions that must be demonstrated by members of the home healthcare interprofessional team.

Professional Dispositions

Professional dispositions are related to the varied concepts of ethics and ethical behavior. They consist of "beliefs, virtues, values, and ethics addressing qualities of character, intellect, and care," and these "dispositions will be manifested in practice and require sophisticated judgment in application" [8]. The display of professional dispositions is paramount when providing quality home healthcare services to clients who are older. Working as a skilled healthcare professional in this setting requires more than having the knowledge and skills of a specific profession or discipline. The healthcare professional must demonstrate qualities, attitudes, and ethical behaviors that will facilitate a positive healthcare environment within the client's home. Health-related services are generally provided by an interprofessional team of diverse disciplines, and each individual discipline and its healthcare personnel are guided by a code of ethics, standards of conduct, or professional principles. Despite each profession having its own code of ethical principles and standards, many of the professional dispositions in healthcare are shared among the varied disciplines. The shared professional dispositions discussed in this chapter comprise what are referred to as the "Three Cs of Professionalism": commitment to competence, commitment to conduct, and commitment to confidentiality (see Fig. 2.1). These three commitments are reflective of each profession's expectation of ethical responsibility and ethical behavior. The three Cs are central to providing quality professional services. They are also hallmarks of professionalism in healthcare professionals.

Commitment to Competence

Receiving care in the home setting requires a certain level of trust between the client and interprofessional healthcare team. Clients are compelled to trust that each healthcare provider that enters the home is knowledgeable of the services provided and that those services are safe and beneficial to their overall health. Clients are also trusting that healthcare providers are honest and upfront about their level of professional competence. Professional competence is rooted in the ethical standards of beneficence, reliability, and transparency and allows the healthcare personnel to

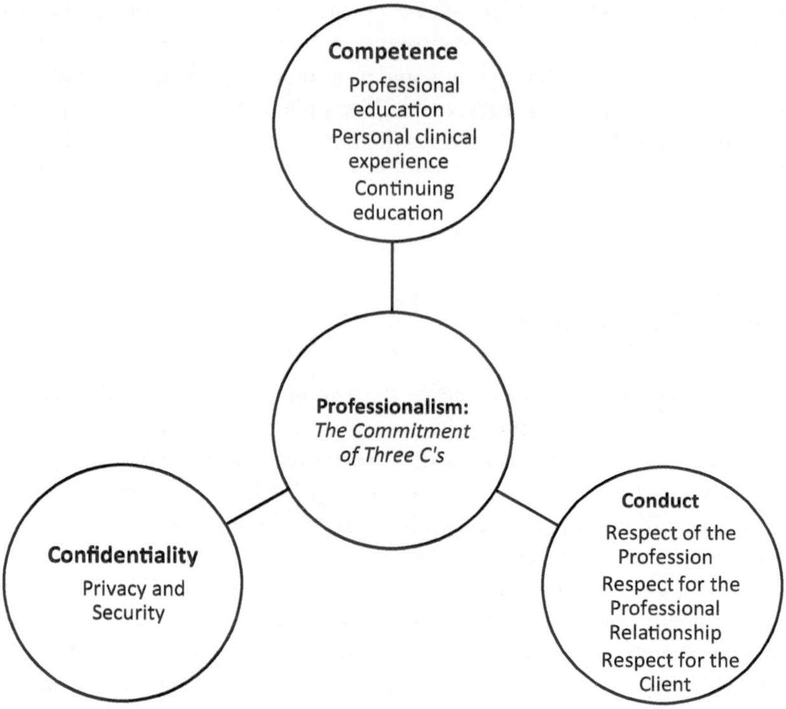

Fig. 2.1 Professionalism: the commitment of three Cs

adequately and sufficiently inform the client of services rendered. Beneficence is an ethical principle that "requires taking action to benefit others—in other words, to promote good, to prevent harm, and to remove harm" [9], whereas reliability is a standard that "ensures clients receive safe, evidenced-based intervention that improves the client's health outcomes" [10]. Transparency is the ethical expectation of providing information that is accurate, accessible, and on a level that the client and caregivers can understand [11]. These ethical standards and principles are interdependent and significant to the quality of home care services provided to clients who are older. The healthcare system and its processes are complex, and older adults may experience more difficulty in knowing, accessing, and managing the type of care, services, and resources they may need [12]. The ethical principles and standards of beneficence, reliability, and transparency reinforce for clients the provider's level of competence, use of sound judgment, and trust that the services rendered are beneficial, safe, and necessary.

Competence and professionalism go hand in hand. "Being professional is the process of obtaining specialized knowledge, skills, attitudes, values, norms and behaviors required to play a role in a profession" [4]. In the authors' view, competence is the process of maintaining or enhancing knowledge, skills, attitudes, values, norms, and behaviors that guide evidence-based practice and clinical decisions. Competency in one's profession is "an ongoing, lifelong process. It begins with your professional education, nurtured and applied in clinical fieldwork experiences, and enhanced through on-the-job experiences that may include further independent study, attendance at continuing education courses, and participation in the supervision process, as well as observing and learning from peers" [13]. Due to the constant changes within the healthcare system, these activities are essential in maintaining competency and providing quality healthcare services throughout the provision of care [13, 14].

Commitment to Conduct

Conduct is another important professional disposition to consider when providing home services to clients who are older. It has been asserted that "a central theme to professionalism involves understanding the formal and informal expectations of conduct associated with the health profession" [14]. Once this expectation of conduct and professional behavior is understood by healthcare providers, they can be effective in providing purposeful and therapeutic services. One quality of conduct that is paramount in the provision of home care services is respect. Interprofessional team members must have respect for the healthcare profession and each discipline of the interprofessional team. There must be respect for the professional relationship between the client and healthcare personnel and, most importantly, respect for the client.

Respect for the Profession

Members of the interprofessional team are representatives of the healthcare profession and their individual discipline. In doing so, the healthcare provider has a duty to represent the profession with veracity by providing accurate, objective, and comprehensive information [9]. This is a key aspect of communicating openly and honestly with clients, both in writing and verbally, to ensure proper education and information. No matter the healthcare setting, whether in a hospital or in a client's home, providers are expected to demonstrate professional behaviors and present themselves in a professional manner. Their behaviors should reflect the values and beliefs held by the profession [13]. Not only does professionalism require a duty of veracity in the representation of the health profession, but it also entails an expectation of professional presentation. Home care may appear to be a more relaxed care setting than the traditional facility setting; however, it is important for the provider to always present as a professional. "In presenting oneself as a professional, consideration must also be given to the provider's attire and appearance to ensure the trust and respect of the client. Professional presentation often communicates to others several indirect messages such as the attitude and competency of the healthcare professional, as well as the level of care or quality of services to be provided. First impressions count, and while it may be true that what a person knows is more important than how he or she looks, the reality is that people form opinions about individuals they meet based on appearances" [13].

Respect for the Professional Relationship

Another important aspect of professional conduct is respect for the professional relationship between the client and the healthcare provider. Providing care to the older population in the home setting has its challenges and limitations. "Factors that contribute to the challenges older individuals face in the home include limited interaction times with the healthcare professionals, and poor communication" [12]. The time used for the client and provider to develop relationships and interact is often limited to the duration allotted for home care services. This limits the opportunities available for the clients to interact with the healthcare provider beyond their scheduled treatment times. Also, "communication is the foundation of all successful relationships, whether it is with family and friends or colleagues and patients" [13], and communication barriers faced by some individuals in this population, such as hearing impairments, visual impairments, and language barriers, can lead to misunderstandings and mistrust. Therefore, special attention is given to the client-provider's professional relationship, interaction, and communication when considering professionalism in the home care setting.

When providing home care, the healthcare providers must know it is important to connect with the client, establish a positive rapport, and work as a collaborative unit. The professional relationship is the basis for building a productive and effective therapeutic relationship. When properly established, this relationship contributes to the client's overall health outcome [13]. Actions of professionalism that contribute to and enhance the professional relationship between the client and healthcare provider include respecting the client's dignity, interests, and goals; acting in a trustworthy manner by providing accurate and reliable information; exhibiting empathic concern about the welfare and well-being of the client; providing justifiable and compassionate service; and communicating openly and on the level of the client's understanding.

Respecting the Client

When providing in-home care, great consideration must be taken to respect the clients, their home environments, and their rights as patients. As with providing care in a healthcare facility, clients receiving care in the home care setting possess certain rights. Clients are entitled to know their health-related rights, to receive an explanation of these rights, and to be supported in exercising their rights. One of these rights includes the right to autonomy, being able to make their own decisions about their medical care without the influence of others. Under the spectrum of autonomy, healthcare professionals should "respect the right of the person to self-determination, privacy, confidentiality, and consent" [9], as well as "treat the client according to their wishes within the accepted standards of care while protecting client confidential information" [13].

Commitment to Confidentiality

The remaining professional disposition commonly shared among various healthcare professionals is a commitment to confidentiality. Clients receiving health-related services possess certain rights as stipulated by local, state, and federal laws and regulations. One important right to enforce in the provision of home care services is the right to privacy and confidentiality. In the healthcare realm, confidentiality refers to the protection of the client's health information. It is an extension of the concept of client privacy which indicates the client has control over and exerts authorization for the utilization of protected health information (PHI). PHI is any information used to identify the client and any health-related services received and may include the client's demographic information, medical records, condition or diagnosis, treatment services, or progress. Confidentiality of PHI is one of several mandates of the Health Insurance Portability and Accountability Act of 1996 (HIPAA). This act serves to improve the effectiveness of quality healthcare services and is the foundation to maintaining client confidentiality and privacy. According to the Centers for Disease Control and Prevention (CDC), HIPAA is a federal law that restricted access to an individual's sensitive medical information and required the development and enforcement of standards that protect patient health information. The US Department of Health and Human Services issued the HIPAA Privacy Law to implement the standards of the HIPAA act and to specifically address the use and disclosure of PHI [15]. The Department issued an equally important Security Rule:

> While the HIPAA Privacy Rule safeguards PHI, the Security Rule protects a subset of information covered by the Privacy Rule. This subset is all individually identifiable health information a covered entity creates, receives, maintains, or transmits in electronic form. This information is called electronic protected health information, or *e-PHI*. The Security Rule does not apply to PHI transmitted orally or in writing [15]

When providing services in the home, the healthcare professional must maintain a commitment to confidentiality through compliance with HIPAA that requires the client's knowledge and consent of the disclosure of sensitive or private medical information and the safeguarding of the client's PHI. Failure to comply with these standards is considered a violation of HIPAA. The delivery of healthcare services provided within the home environment potentially exposes the client to the loss of confidentiality and complicates HIPAA compliance for home care professionals. It is likely these services may be provided to the client in the presence of other individuals such as family, friends, neighbors, clergy, and other healthcare professionals. In this digital age, it is common for the use of portable electronic devices such as laptops, tablets, and cellular phones as a medium to complete documentation of services. As a result, the healthcare professional may unintentionally and inadvertently share PHI through communications overheard or casual conversations in the home, unsecure documents or portable devices, or unsecure, unencrypted Internet networks. To mitigate and minimize the risk of breaching confidentiality and privacy, healthcare professionals must always be cognizant of their professionalism and possess a commitment to HIPAA compliance and client confidentiality in the delivery of healthcare and provision of quality home care services. "This involves forming collaborative relationships with recipients and their caregivers in setting goals and priorities; providing full disclosure of the benefits, respecting the recipient's right to refuse services; ensuring confidentiality and the right to privacy are respected and maintained; and maintaining the confidentiality of all communications" [13]. In maintaining client confidentiality, certain methods are taken to safeguard any health-related information related to the client or information that discloses the identity of the client. See Box 2.1 for common mistakes home care workers should avoid. Mindful considerations of these actions on a day-to-day basis will result in service delivery that is respectful of clients' right to privacy and confidentiality [16]. These common mistakes can undermine efforts to build rapport and trust with clients and jeopardize professional licensure or certification.

Box 2.1: Common Mistakes Home Care Workers Should Avoid [16]

(a) *Noncompliance with State HIPAA Laws.* Many organizations ensure compliance with HIPAA regulations at the federal level. Organizations and employees must also follow HIPAA regulations at the state level.
(b) *Not Informing Patients.* Patients must be informed of their rights to privacy as it relates to their health information.
(c) *Improperly Disclosing Information.* It is easy to accidentally disclose confidential patient information in a casual conversation. Employees should only discuss patient information with the clients themselves or their authorized representatives.
(d) *Using Non-encrypted Networks to Store or Transmit Health Information.* Agency staff must be mindful of storing and transmitting PHI only through networks that have been secured with the proper encryption.
(e) *Unsecured Records.* Failing to physically secure information. Whether it is keeping passwords in plain sight, not keeping a watchful eye on small portable devices that can easily be lost or stolen, or losing paperwork when transporting it between the patient's home and agency, home care employees must securely store paperwork, passwords, and data.
(f) *Improper Disposal of Patient Records.* Employees must shred or destroy all patient health information and medical records once they are no longer of use or expired. Employees cannot throw away any documents or hard drives with patient information on them.

(continued)

Box 2.1 (continued)

(g) *Accessing PHI Through Personal Devices.* Employees should not do work on personal devices that may lack the appropriate password protection or access to properly secured networks. They also should not allow others access to any device used for work purposes.

(h) *Improperly Releasing Information.* Before releasing patient information to anyone, agencies and providers must confirm that patients have current HIPAA authorization forms on file. Releasing patient data even 1 day after a form has expired can result in a HIPAA violation.

(i) *Lost or Stolen Devices.* Theft of PHI through lost or stolen devices can easily result in HIPAA fines and penalties. Mobile devices are the most vulnerable to theft because of their size; therefore, agencies must employ strategies such as password protection, encryption, and remote wiping to prevent unauthorized access to patient-specific information on devices.

(j) *Illegally Accessing Patient Files Within the Workplace.* Employees should never access patient information unless they have been specifically authorized to do so.

Clinical Documentation

Clinical documentation is necessary for a variety of reasons. Good clinical documentation is a critical means of recording essential clinical information about patient care, interprofessional communication, reimbursement, and risk management. As clinical documentation standards evolve, more health agencies and providers are transitioning to electronic health records (EHR) to enhance documentation efficiency. EHRs are computer-created medical records. However, specific minimum standards are expected for both paper records and EHRs. Clinical documentation is particularly important when caring for patients who are older within the home environment. These individuals are often deemed as *vulnerable* due to comorbidities and medical fragility.

Elements of Quality Clinical Documentation

Clinical documentation communicates what, when, why, where, and how clinical care is delivered to patients. Clinical documentation varies depending on the context (e.g., an initial evaluation differs from a treatment progress note). *Initial or primary patient documentation* may comprise demographics, psychosocial history, medical history, and review of examination results (e.g., systems review, tests or measures, level of function, medications, lab results, etc.). *Evaluative documentation* is used to determine the appropriate diagnosis, impairments or functional limitations, prognosis, plan of care including SMART functional goals, and treatment interventions required for skilled care. The plan of care must be congruent with the patient's clinical needs. Informed consent, an integral element of clinical documentation, should be secured and documented prior to the provision of services [17]. *Progress documentation* typically provides details about patients' response to treatment and their progress toward functional goals. Progress documentation provides justification for ongoing treatment in the context of medical necessity or for changes to the goals or care plan. Progress documentation also encompasses recommendations for reassessments [18]. *Concluding documentation* typically is referred to as a discharge summary or closing summary. These documents typically include dates of service, diagnoses, skilled services provided, progress toward goals and outcomes, functional status at discharge, evidence of patient education, justification for discharge, treatment complications and comorbidities, and recommendations for continuity of care [19]. Clinical documentation can serve as a pathway for communication between multiple healthcare practitioners, thus fostering interprofessional communication. All clinical contacts (including phone calls) should be documented, signed, and dated. The time or duration of the service contact should also be indicated.

Payment for Services

Clinical documentation should be conducted ethically. Any billing submitted for reimbursement should be accurate, justifiable, and well-supported by clinical documentation. The healthcare provider should become familiar with the expectations of the payer in order to meet the payer's documentation requirements. Regarding in-home health for older patients, Medicare is commonly the payer with specific requirements, e.g., documentation of medical necessity, progression, and timed interventions. Documentation is commonly provided using the Outcome and Assessment Information Set (OASIS) in home health [20]. OASIS contains items the Centers for Medicare and Medicaid developed to measure patient outcomes and determine agency reimbursement. These items include Health Insurance Prospective Payment System (HIPPS) rate codes, which represent specific sets of patient characteristics (or case-mix groups) on which payment determinations are made under several prospective payment systems; sociodemographic variables; information on the patient home environment and informal caregivers; health status, including diagnosis codes; functional status; psychosocial status; and health service utilization (emergent care or hospital admission, or both) [21]. The OASIS assessments are required of all home health agencies certified to accept Medicare and Medicaid payments. Additionally, Medicare patients' clinical notes must illustrate that skilled services are being provided, the patient is progressing continuously as a result of the services, and the services are reasonable and medically necessary. When patients are not progressing toward their goals, documentation must show appropriate modifications in the intervention or identification of any problems that may impede progress and impact outcomes. It is essential to include the patient's homebound status in home health [20]. Home health documentation (e.g., initial patient assessments and subsequent assessments) is used to support the patient's homebound status and need for skilled care [22].

Risk Management

Ethical documentation of clinical services minimizes a variety of risks in the home care milieu. It provides support against malpractice claims or potential lawsuits. It serves as a protection for all parties involved providing a permanent account of the episode of care as it evolved, serving as a reference for quality assurance, and substantiating compliance with appropriate practices and state and federal statutes. Documentation demonstrates whether the standard of practice has been met. Clinical documentation is commonly the primary evidence in a malpractice case; therefore, it is critical that clinical notes are comprehensive, professionally written, and accurate. Any errors in the record should be properly corrected with a single line through the error, followed by the clinician's initials and the date. Any amendments to the record should be clearly identified as such, signed by the provider and dated. Poor documentation may result in the loss of the provider's professional license [23].

It is always beneficial to review documentation for errors or oversights. Professional documentation should be free from spelling, grammar, and punctuation errors. The provider should use only approved abbreviations. All clinical documentation should be legible, signed, and dated. Clinical documentation should also include the credentials of the provider. All student documentation should be cosigned by the appropriate practitioner, as required by the payer or state licensure board or both [18]. Clinical documentation is typically more accurate and comprehensive when completed at the time of service or as soon as possible after care is provided [20]. Incident reporting is particularly important when providing care to patients who are older. Patient accidents or injuries or visible scarring or marks should be promptly documented and communicated to the medical authority and other members of the interprofessional team. The report should document the presence of witnesses who may have knowledge of the scarring or marks and include statements from witnesses. Statements from the patient should also be recorded. In instances of suspected abuse or neglect, adult protective services or law enforcement should be contacted [23]. Maltreatment and abuse of older adults is discussed in more detail in the following session.

Maltreatment or Abuse of Older Adults

Maltreatment or abuse of older adults is a growing problem, made even more severe by the challenges involved in identifying and reporting such abuse. Older adults are often more susceptible to various forms of abuse. Many older adults depend on others to meet their most basic needs. Their mistreatment can be by family members, strangers, healthcare providers, caregivers, friends, or "trusted others." Abuse is an intentional act or failure to act that causes or creates a risk of harm to an older adult. An older adult is someone who is age 60 or older [24].

Types of Maltreatment or Abuse of Older Adults

There are several common forms of abuse. *Verbal abuse* is the use of words to assault, dominate, ridicule, manipulate, or degrade another person and negatively impact the person's psychological health. *Physical abuse* is physical force to inflict injury, pain, or death. *Neglect* is failure to protect an older adult or to meet the individual's essential needs. These needs include food, water, shelter, clothing, hygiene, or medical care. *Sexual abuse* is forcing a person to engage in sexual interactions. *Emotional/psychological abuse* is behaviors that harm a person's mental or emotional well-being. *Financial exploitation* is unauthorized or improper use of an older adult's resources to the disadvantage of the person or the profit or benefit of other persons. *Abandonment* is when a person assumes responsibility for providing care to an individual who is older but then deserts or willfully neglects that individual [24]. Abuse of older adults can be the result of risk factors unique to the patient who is older, the caregiver, and the environment. Patient factors may include functional dependence, disability, poor physical health, cognitive impairment, poor mental health, low income or socioeconomic status, gender, age, financial dependence, or race or ethnicity. Caregiver factors may include mental illness, substance abuse, and abuser dependency. Environmental factors include care milieu, staffing problems, lack of qualified staff, staff burnout, and stressful working conditions [25].

Signs of Maltreatment or Abuse of Older Adults

Any of the following signs, solely, may not substantiate intentional or willful maltreatment or abuse. Signs of maltreatment or abuse are unique to the patient, caregiver, or environment. Patient: confusion or delirium, dehydration, malnutrition, decayed teeth, overgrown nails, matted hair, infested hair, overmedication or undermedication or mis-medication, unexplained weight loss, or pressure ulcers. Caregiver: missing or absent, living in significantly better conditions than the person who is older despite living in the same residence, more focused on the cost of care than the needs of the patient (especially when the patient is financially stable), appears overburdened or resentful of caregiving duties, withholds services to punish or discipline, or disregard of calls for assistance. Environment: Residence is poorly maintained, unsafe, or unclean, lacks heating or cooling, lacks appropriate food and hydration, has a foul odor, is infested with vermin or bugs, or lacks prescribed assistive devices that were previously present in the home [26].

Reporting Maltreatment or Abuse of Older Adults

Every state has laws pertaining to the maltreatment of older adults with variations in language and applicability. The laws in most states require "helping professions" such as healthcare providers to report suspected abuse or neglect. The provider may report by contacting any or a combination of the following:

- Law enforcement at a designated emergency number (if abuse is life-threatening or there is the possibility of a crime).
- Adult protective services.
- Licensing board of a skilled nursing facility, group home, or other geriatric center or service facility.
- Ombudsman (if abuse is in a facility).
- Older persons abuse hotlines.
- Licensing board of healthcare provider suspected of maltreatment or abuse.

If appropriate, the healthcare provider may need to refer the individual to a domestic violence or sexual assault service organization. The onus is not on the healthcare provider to prove that maltreatment or abuse is occurring. The appropriate authority will conduct their investigation and make such determination [27].

Cross-Cultural Communication

Effective cross-cultural communication is essential to achieving positive healthcare outcomes with patients who are older. Thus, efforts should be taken to reduce or eliminate obstacles that impede cross-cultural communication while providing care within the home setting. It is also important that the models of cross-cultural communication guide the interactions with individuals whose cultures are different from the professionals.

Cross-cultural communication is the process of sending and receiving messages between people whose cultural background could lead them to interpret verbal and nonverbal signs differently. It refers to an exchange of information and meaning between individuals or groups from different backgrounds. Different cultures communicate differently. Factors affecting interactions between diverse cultures include history, religion, family, gender roles, education, values, and attitudes. Cultural differences can often result in misunderstandings [28]. The prudent healthcare provider will devote time to asking questions about the aforementioned factors. Many of these factors will influence the patient-provider relationship, the patient's comfort level while receiving care within the home setting, and the patient's success in attaining care goals.

Cross-cultural communication is important at every phase of care (e.g., informed consent, preliminary information gathering, evaluation and reassessment, progress reporting, discharge, aftercare, and follow-up services). Communication can be verbal (e.g., words, voice tone, vocal characteristics) or nonverbal (e.g., facial expressions, eye contact, proximity, gestures, posture, touch, physiological changes, and personal appearance) [29].

Effective cross-cultural communication begins with the provider personally assessing cultural biases and values. It is particularly important that providers acknowledge that cultural differences do exist between themselves and their patients. These differences should never be discounted or minimized. The healthcare provider should strive to be a reflective practitioner. *Reflective practice* is the ability to reflect on personal actions and to take a critical stance or attitude toward one's own practices and that of one's peers. Reflective practice comprises engaging in continuous adaptation and learning and reflecting on the past to shape the future. Reflective practitioners consciously examine their emotions, experiences, actions, and responses [30].

Healthcare providers who struggle to become culturally competent in their communication with patients should be mindful of being ethnocentrism or stereotyping [31]. Ethnocentrism is the belief in the superiority of one's own ethnic group. Stereotyping involves a standardized picture of a group that represents an oversimplified opinion or prejudiced attitude. Stereotyping may also include generalizing based on misperceptions, discrimination, or biases about a person's background or health beliefs [32]. Additional strategies for effective cross-cultural communication include researching the patient's culture to learn about communication styles. This research can inform about words and actions that are perceived as being courteous as well as strategies for keeping communication simple and avoiding slang, jargon, and taboo topics. The primary goal of effective cross-cultural communication is to increase patient understanding, establish rapport and trust, and improve health outcomes.

Cross-Cultural Communication Differences

To better assist individuals in appreciating communication differences among ethnic cultural groups, anthropologist Edward T. Hall coined the terms "low-context" and "high-context" [33]. High-context cultures are those in which the rules of communication are primarily transmitted through the use of contextual elements or indirect communication. Japan, Arab countries, Korea, and Latin America are examples of high-context cultures. High-context cultures rely less on words and more on intuition, body language, a person's status, and tone of voice. Thus, information may not be explicitly stated. In low-context cultures, information is communicated primarily through language; rules are explicitly spelled out and verbal communication is more direct. The USA and most European countries are examples of low-context cultures. People in low-context cultures generally do not pay much attention to body language, tone of voice, or a person's status. These contextual concepts are broad descriptions of differences in communication styles between cultures. Knowing these differences can be helpful when learning to communicate across ethnic cultures with patients who are older.

Effective communication can help build satisfying relationships with older patients. It can strengthen the patient-provider relationship, improve health outcomes, help prevent medical errors, and maximize limited interaction time. A key communication tip that can help facilitate successful interactions with older persons is to always speak to them adult-to-adult. Additionally, it is important to make the older patient feel comfortable by acknowledging both verbal and nonverbal communication; avoiding rushing or pressuring the older adult to speak; speaking clearly and slowly; accommodating for hearing, visual, and cognitive deficits; recognizing cultural differences; providing a summary of major points, using appropriate digital technology; and including the caregiver when necessary [34].

Cross-Cultural Communication Models

Some cross-cultural communication models include LEARN, RESPECT, and the iceberg model. These models are geared toward providing guidance on effective ways of communicating across cultures.

LEARN Model: Skills for Clinical Care [35–37]

- L – listen to the patient
- E – elicit patients' health beliefs
- A – assess potential problems that may have an impact on health behaviors.
- R – recommend a treatment plan.
- N – negotiate a mutually agreed-on treatment plan

RESPECT MODEL: Building Cross-Cultural Trust [37, 38].

- R – rapport
  - Connect on a social level.
  - Seek the patient's point of view.
  - Consciously attempt to suspend judgment.
  - Recognize and avoid making assumptions.
- E – empathy
  - Remember that the patient has come to you for help.
  - Seek out and understand the patient's rationale for his or her behaviors or illness
  - Verbally acknowledge and legitimize the patient's feelings.
- S – support
  - Ask about and try to understand barriers to care and compliance
  - Help the patient overcome barriers.
  - Involve family members if appropriate.
  - Reassure the patient you are and will be available to help.

- P – partnership
  - Be flexible with regard to issues of control.
  - Negotiate roles when necessary.
  - Stress that you will be working together to address medical problems.
- E – explanations
  - Check often for understanding.
  - Use verbal clarification techniques.
- C – cultural competence (humility and responsibility)
  - Respect the patient's culture and beliefs.
  - Understand that ethnic or cultural stereotypes may identify the patient's view of you.
  - Be aware of your own biases and preconceptions.
  - Know your limitations in addressing medical issues across cultures.
  - Understand your personal style and recognize when it may not be working with a given patient.
- T – trust
  - Self-disclosure may be an issue for some patients who are not accustomed to Western medical approaches
  - Take the necessary time and consciously work to establish trust

Iceberg Model

- The *cultural iceberg* has two parts: visible conscious aspects and unseen unconscious aspects. The iceberg model [33] can be described as 10% "above the surface" (behaviors, traditions, and customs that are explicitly learned and conscious, objective knowledge that is easily changed) and 90% "deep below the surface" (core values, priorities, attitudes, beliefs, and assumptions that are implicitly learned and unconscious subjective knowledge that is difficult to change). This model teaches professionals that they cannot judge a culture based only on what is visible to the eye. As responsible interprofessional team members, each professional must take the time to get to know and engage with their patients from the patients' cultural perspectives. Only by doing so can professionals uncover the values and beliefs that underlie their existence. When professionals appreciate and understand the culture of older patients, they can tailor the treatment or care plan to meet their needs. Although professionals cannot be an expert in all cultural norms and practices, always being respectful, asking questions, and practicing cultural humility can strengthen patient-provider relationships.

Chapter Summary

Factors such as the COVID-19 pandemic, shifts in the older population distribution, and increasing healthcare costs have contributed to an increasing tendency for health service provision in the home setting [4]. In the facility environment, services provided are generally based on clients' subjective report of their needs, resources, and relationships within the home. In contrast, the home environment exposes clients' most intimate selves, their physical home environment and interactions with family members, and their actual functional performance. Unique challenges are faced by healthcare providers in the home care environment, and one of these challenges is professionalism. [4]. Professionalism is key in ensuring clients receive adequate and acceptable care within the delicate setting of the home without loss of dignity, autonomy, or confidentiality. This chapter emphasizes the importance of professionalism as well as the correlation between this very important concept and the provision of quality home care services to patients who are older.

When discussing professional ethics of healthcare providers in the home setting, consideration must be given to clinical documentation, maltreatment and abuse, and cross-cultural communication. Clinical documentation must meet professional and organizational standards of care, regulatory requirements, and reimbursement requirements. Clinical documentation is the core of professional accountability and a means for interprofessional communication.

Maltreatment or abuse of older adults can occur in various forms, including neglect, physical abuse, sexual abuse, emotional or psychological abuse, financial exploitation, and abandonment. The risk factors and signs may involve the victim, the caregiver, and the environment. The healthcare provider is obligated to report maltreatment and abuse of older adults. Effective cross-cultural communication is essential to achieve positive healthcare outcomes. Developing cross-cultural communication skills, identifying differences among cultural groups, and utilizing a cross-cultural communication model can help reduce or eliminate obstacles that impede cross-cultural communication when working with patients who are older in the home setting.

Discussion Questions

1. Define professionalism and explain its importance throughout the provision of home care services for older adults.
2. What are some of the shared professional dispositions among the interprofessional team discussed in this chapter for healthcare personnel in the provision of home care services?
3. Why is good clinical documentation necessary in healthcare?
4. Discuss three models that can be used to facilitate cross-cultural communication in healthcare for older adults.

Multiple Choice Questions

1. Which of the following are three aspects of professional conduct as discussed in this chapter?
   (a) Respect for the client
   (b) Respect for the profession
   (c) Respect for the professional relationship
   (d) All of the above
2. All members of the interprofessional team who provide home care services to older adults are expected to abide by certain ethical expectations and standards as dictated by their individual profession.
   (a) True
   (b) False
3. The Healthcare Insurance Portability and Accountability Act of 1996 is a federal law that safeguards the privacy and security of patient information except for which of the following?
   (a) Medical diagnosis or condition
   (b) Treatment services and progress
   (c) Employment records
   (d) Demographic Information
4. In clinical documentation, what is the *most* important characteristic of a patient goal? The goal is…
   (a) Concise
   (b) Functional
   (c) Flexible
   (d) Idealistic
5. A therapist meets with the wife of a 70-year-old man. The wife informs the therapist that her husband is receiving home health services following a total hip replacement. The client is concerned that her husband is not receiving adequate care because he appears weaker and fearful. She shares that he has developed bed sores and is becoming increasingly withdrawn. The client would like to change to another home care agency. How should the therapist proceed?
   (a) Honor the client's self-determination and assist her in identifying another home care agency.
   (b) Assess further for potential abuse of older adults to determine if a report is required.
   (c) Inform the client a report is mandated and provide verbal and written report to both law enforcement and the local ombudsman.
   (d) Consult with colleagues to determine if this information rises to the level of reasonable suspicion of abuse.

References

1. Social Security Administration. (2014, January 1). *Calculators: Life expectancy*. Retrieved September 18, 2014 from http://www.ssa.gov/planners/lifeexpectancy.htm
2. Qualls, S. H., & Zarit, S. (Eds.). (2009). *Aging families and caregiving*. Wiley.
3. Resnick, B. (2013). *Settings for care*. Retrieved September 15, 2013, from http://www.merckmanuals.com/home/older-people%E2%80%99s-health-issues/provision-of-care-to-older-people/settings-for-care
4. Fatemi, N. L., Moonaghi, H. K., & Heydari, A. (2018). Exploration of nurses' perception about professionalism in home care nursing in Iran: A qualitative study. *Electronic Physician, 10*(5), 6803–6811. https://doi.org/10.19082/6803
5. Cornett, B. (2006). A principal calling: Professionalism and health care services. *Journal of Communication Disorders, 39*(4), 301–309. https://doi.org/10.1016/j.jcomdis.2006.02.005
6. Brehm, B., Breen, P., Brown, B., Long, L., Smith, R., Wall, A., & Warren, N. S. (2006). An interdisciplinary approach to introducing professionalism. *American Journal of Pharmaceutical Education, 70*(4), 81. https://doi.org/10.5688/aj700481
7. Hammer, D., et al. (2012). Defining and measuring the construct of interprofessional professionalism. *Journal of Allied Health, 41*(2), e49–e53.
8. Sockett, H. (2006). Character, rules, and relations. In *Teacher dispositions: Building a teacher education framework of moral standards* (pp. 9–25).
9. American Occupational Therapy Association. (2020). Occupational therapy practice framework (4th ed.). *American Journal of Occupational Therapy* 74 (Supplement_2) :7412410010p1–7412410010, p. 87.doi: https://doi.org/10.5014/ajot.2020.74S2001.
10. Pronovost, P. J., Berenholtz, S. M., Goeschel, C. A., Needham, D. M., Sexton, J. B., Thompson, D. A., et al. (2006). Creating high reliability in health care organizations. *Health Services Research, 41*(4p2), 1599–1617.
11. Oettgen, Peter. (n.d.). *Transparency in healthcare: Achieving clarity in healthcare through transparent reporting of clinical data*. EBSCO Health: DynaMed Plus https://www.ebsco.com/sites/g/files/nabnos191/files/acquiadam-assets/66751087.pdf
12. Gong, N., Meng, Y., Hu, Q., et al. (2002). Obstacles to access to community care in urban senior-only households: A qualitative study. *BMC Geriatrics, 22*, 122. https://doi.org/10.1186/s12877-022-02816-y
13. Davis, L., & Rosee, M. (2015). *Occupational therapy student to clinician: Making the transition*. Slack, Incorporated. Thorofare.
14. Garman, A. N., Evans, R., Krause, M. K., & Anfossi, J. (2006). Professionalism. *Journal of Healthcare Management, 51*(4), 219.
15. Centers for Disease and Control. (2022). *Health insurance portability and accountability act of 1996*. https://www.cdc.gov/phlp/publications/topic/hipaa.html
16. Moore, W., & Frye, S. (2019). Review of HIPAA, part 1: History, protected health information, and privacy and security rules. *Journal of Nuclear Medicine Technology, 47*(4), 269–272. https://doi.org/10.2967/jnmt.119.227819
17. *Elements of Documentation Within the Patient/Client Management Model*. (2018, January 31). APTA. https://www.apta.org/your-practice/documentation/defensible-documentation/elements-within-the-patientclient-management-model
18. *Documentation in Health Care*. (n.d.). American Speech-Language-Hearing Association. https://www.asha.org/practice-portal/professional-issues/documentation-in-health-care/
19. Syed, S. (2017, November 5). *Clinical documentation | How to document medical information well*. Onthewards. https://onthewards.org/how-to-document-well/
20. Sims, P. B. (2016). *Launch into home health physical therapy*.
21. Home Health Outcome and Assessment Information Set | ResDAC. (n.d.). Resdac.org. https://resdac.org/cms-data/files/oasis
22. *Determining Homebound*. (n.d.). *CGS Medicare*. Retrieved April 1, 2023, from https://www.cgsmedicare.com

23. Documentation: Risk Management. (2019, December 18). APTA. https://www.apta.org/your-practice/documentation/defensible-documentation/risk-management
24. Uniform definitions and recommended core data elements for use in elder abuse surveillance. Version 1.0. (n.d.). Stacks.cdc.gov. https://stacks.cdc.gov/view/cdc/37909
25. Pillemer, K., Burnes, D., Riffin, C., & Lachs, M. S. (2016). Elder abuse: Global situation, risk factors, and prevention strategies. *The Gerontologist, 56*(Suppl 2), S194–S205. https://doi.org/10.1093/geront/gnw004
26. National Institute on Aging. (n.d.) *Spotting the signs of elder abuse*. National Institute on Aging. https://www.nia.nih.gov/health/infographics/spotting-signs-elder-abuse
27. Digital Communications Division (DCD). (2015, June 8). *How do I report elder abuse or abuse of an older person or senior?* HHS.gov. https://www.hhs.gov/answers/programs-for-families-and-children/how-do-i-report-elder-abuse/index.html
28. Prabhakaran, Kavitha. (2015). *Cross culture communication*. https://doi.org/10.13140/RG.2.2.32617.44649.
29. University of St Augustine. (2020, February 26). *The importance of effective communication in nursing*. University of St. Augustine for Health Sciences. https://www.usa.edu/blog/communication-in-nursing/
30. Taylor, S. P., Nicolle, C., & Maguire, M. (2013). Cross-cultural communication barriers in health care. *Nursing Standard, 27*(31), 35–43. https://doi.org/10.7748/ns2013.04.27.31.35.e7040
31. Kumar, D. (n.d.). *Cross-cultural communication and negotiation – A conceptual framework*. Www.academia.edu. Retrieved December 31, 2022, from https://www.academia.edu/16058728/Cross_Cultural_Communication_and_Negotiation_A_Conceptual_Framework
32. 7.1: *Ethnocentrism and Stereotypes*. (2020, March 31). *Social Sci LibreTexts*. https://socialsci.libretexts.org/Courses/Butte_College/Exploring_Intercultural_Communication_(Grothe)/07%3A_Barriers_to_Intercultural_Communication/7.01%3A_Ethnocentrism_and_Stereotypes
33. Hall, E. T. (1976). *Beyond culture*. Anchor Books. Excerpts available at https://www.academia.edu/56977386/Beyond_Culture_Edward_T_Hall
34. National Institute on Aging. (2023, January 25). *Talking with your older patients*. National Institute on Aging. https://www.nia.nih.gov/health/talking-your-older-patients.
35. Berlin, E. A., & Fowkes, W. C., Jr. (1983 Dec). A teaching framework for cross-cultural health care. Application in family practice. *The Western Journal of Medicine, 139*(6), 934–938.
36. Ladha, T., Zubairi, M., Hunter, A., Audcent, T., & Johnstone, J. (2018). Cross-cultural communication: Tools for working with families and children. *Paediatrics & Child Health, 23*(1), 66–69. https://doi.org/10.1093/pch/pxx126
37. Welch, M. (1998). *Enhancing awareness and improving cultural competence in health care. A partnership guide for teaching diversity and cross-cultural concepts in health professional training*. University of California at San Francisco.
38. Mostow, C., Crosson, J., Gordon, S., Chapman, S., Gonzalez, P., Hardt, E., Delgado, L., James, T., & David, M. (2010). Treating and precepting with RESPECT: A relational model addressing race, ethnicity, and culture in medical training. *Journal of General Internal Medicine, 25*(S2), 146–154. https://doi.org/10.1007/s11606-010-1274-4

Chapter 3
Patient-Client and Family Caregiver Considerations

Gilaine Nettles, Mary-Anne Joseph, and Jared Rehm

Learning Objectives

1. Understand historical perspectives pertaining to the value of patient- and family-centered care.
2. Describe ways to improve the home care experience for patients who are older.
3. Articulate the characteristics and responsibilities of family caregivers.
4. Identify challenges faced by family caregivers in home care settings.
5. Articulate quality of life and wellness strategies for patients and family caregivers.
6. Provide examples of patient autonomy and choice making in the home care setting.

Historical Perspectives on Person-Centered Care, Family Caregiving, and Interprofessional Collaboration

Essential to the interprofessional team (IP) approach to quality healthcare is the concept of *patient-centeredness*. The significance of the patient being at the *center* of care delivery has been recognized for many decades. In 2001, the Institute of Medicine released a paper called "Crossing the Quality Chasm: A New Health System for the 21st Century" [1]. The paper underscored the importance of patient-centeredness in improving healthcare systems. Similarly, a few years later, the

Supplementary Information The online version contains supplementary material available at https://doi.org/10.1007/978-3-031-40889-2_3.

G. Nettles (✉) · J. Rehm
Department of Physical Therapy, College of Health Sciences, Alabama State University, Montgomery, AL, USA
e-mail: gnettles@alasu.edu; jrehm@alasu.edu

M.-A. Joseph
Department of Rehabilitation Studies, College of Health Sciences, Alabama State University, Montgomery, AL, USA
e-mail: majoseph@alasu.edu

D. H. Stapleton, S. Bossie (eds.), *Home Care for Older Adults Using Interprofessional Teams*, https://doi.org/10.1007/978-3-031-40889-2_3

Triple Aim framework refocused healthcare providers' attention on the significance of patient-centered care [2].

The Interprofessional Education Collaborative (IPEC) was established in the USA in 2009. Its mission is to prepare healthcare professionals to become collaborative practitioners by implementing interprofessional education in all professional programs. The ultimate goal of interprofessional education and collaboration is to assure patient-centered care. In 2010, the World Health Organization (WHO) released a framework for collaborative practice and interprofessional education. The framework provided guidelines for healthcare professionals to learn from one another, to collaborate in clinical practice, and to effectively develop and implement patient care plans. By cooperating with patients and their families and caregivers, collaborative practitioners build teams that are founded on mutual respect, shared values, and positive communication [3].

In 2011, the interprofessional collaborative panel, composed of six participating professional organizations, united to create the core competency domains for interprofessional collaboration and healthcare delivery. These six professional organizations included the American Association of Colleges of Nursing, the American Association of Colleges of Osteopathic Medicine, the American Association of Colleges of Pharmacy, the American Dental Education Association, the Association of American Medical Colleges, and the Association of Schools and Programs of Public Health. The core competency domains included (1) teams and teamwork, (2) communication, (3) roles and responsibilities, and (4) values and ethics [4]. In 2016, nine new disciplines joined IPEC [5]. The new professions included podiatry, physical therapy, occupational therapy, psychology, veterinary medicine, social work, and physician's assistant education. This new group (the Health Professionals Accreditor Collaborative) further developed the core competencies and expanded the shared vision of achieving quality outcomes in healthcare and improving health equity in population health through collaborative educational learning experiences and practices [5]. This was a positive development for those strongly advocating for more patient-centered healthcare systems.

The Quadruple Aim, published in 2014, evidenced that when IP teams worked collaboratively with patients and families, both patient and provider satisfaction with care increased. Patients reported feeling a part of the team and better connected with healthcare providers. Patients also reported better disease management and better health outcomes [6]. The Quadruple Aim addressed the effects of provider stress, fatigue, and burnout and highlighted the need to enhance providers' healthcare experiences. These improved experiences would impact patients' quality of care and safety, but they would also enhance the care experiences of each IP team member [7].

Additional Federal Reports on Family Caregiving

In 2016, the National Academy of Sciences, Engineering, and Medicine (NASEM) developed an ad hoc committee on family caregiving for older adults. The committee was tasked with the following: (1) investigating the prevalence of family caregiving and the consequences of caregiving on caregivers, (2) exploring existing programs designed to meet the needs of caregivers, and (3) providing recommendations for policies to support caregivers. Similarly, the 2016 NASEM report entitled "Families Caring for an Aging America" provided recommendations for policy changes to better support caregivers' health, economic, and social needs through agencies such as the Centers for Medicare and Medicaid Services, Social Security, and the Department of Veterans Affairs. Such policy changes would propel an awareness of the tremendous demand for caregivers due to the growing older adult population and the diminished supply of trained caregivers.

According to the NASEM report, 72.8 million US residents will be over the age of 65 by 2030. Furthermore, those in their 80 s and older are expected to increase to approximately 37% of the population by 2050 [8]. Without an adequate supply of trained caregivers, this responsibility is increasingly falling on family members. Many family caregivers assume the role by default because no one else is available or willing to provide continuous care for the patient. This special report also revealed that spouses and daughters are likely to be primary caregivers and spend the most time providing care and making caregiving decisions. Secondary caregivers tend to be men who provide intermittent care and often support the primary caregiver.

The Committee of Family Caregiving was established to study trends in caregiving. The committee utilized data and findings from the National Health and Aging Trends Study (NHATS) and the National Study of Caregiving (NSOC) to aid them in compiling a report with recommendations for federal and state agencies. The study surveyed Medicare beneficiaries who were over the age of 65 and needed caregiver assistance with activities of daily living (e.g., toileting, transferring, bathing, dressing, grooming, or continence). More than half of the caregivers in the study were employed and needed the benefit of time off to assist family members. The study exposed the need for more policies and programs to support caregivers and the need for more research to identify strategies for lessening the stress and strain of family caregivers [9]. The COVID-19 pandemic resulted in large numbers of patients requiring medical treatment [10]. With the shelter-in-place requirement and limited hospital access, caregiver burden during the pandemic was exacerbated.

Improving the Home Care Experience of Older Patients

One of the authors of this chapter is particularly grateful for the IP team's role in maximizing her father's home care experience:

My father said that he never wanted to go to a nursing home and he wanted to stay in his home and age in place. Working with the interprofessional team helped me to grant his wishes. In doing so, we had many challenges on a daily basis and it was not always the best situation. But, being at home was better for him than being anywhere else. I am grateful for all of the healthcare providers who guided his home health care. (Gilaine Nettles)

Transforming a home environment into a healthcare environment can be a daunting task. However, members of the IP team are experts at suggesting ways to create a safe and therapeutic environment. For example, physical and occupational therapists can provide low-cost suggestions to increase safety in the home such as installing grab bars, removing throw rugs and clutter, replacing doorknobs with handles, and promoting the use of adaptive equipment. However, some changes can be expensive and more complicated (e.g., adding a fully accessible first-floor bathroom) [11]. In these instances, the IP team should work conjointly with the family to locate trustworthy and affordable contractors. Similarly, home maintenance may become more difficult for older patients, and the cost for maintaining a safe home environment can be quite expensive. Unrepaired floors, steps, and bathroom structures can become safety hazards [12]. The IP team should continuously evaluate the home environment and make necessary recommendations. Team members should link families with appropriate community resources that will promote patient safety and accessibility within the home setting [13].

To maximize the patient's home care experience, IP teams may solicit the support of family members, friends, and other caregivers. Having an established support system can enhance the older patient's level of motivation, compliance, confidence, and satisfaction. A support system is also important when creating opportunities for continuity of care. IP team members can conduct informational sessions with family members and caregivers to facilitate caregiving skill development and appropriate engagement with all healthcare tasks [14].

Health Literacy

As people age, they become more susceptible to health conditions that impact their levels of functioning and their ability to find meaning and purpose in life. For many older adults, this is a period of adjustment. Many older patients struggle to fully understand their health conditions and their new reality as it relates to diminished capacities. Health literacy is useful in helping patients adapt to the biopsychosocial effects of illness and disease. Health literacy is equally beneficial for caregivers. According to the Centers for Disease Control and Prevention (CDC), "personal health literacy is the degree to which individuals have the ability to find, understand, and use information and services to inform health-related decisions and actions for themselves and others" [15]. Approximately 88% of adults in the USA have inadequate levels of health literacy that prevent them from navigating the healthcare system and enhancing their well-being [16]. Only 12% of people living in the USA were found to be proficient in health literacy. The lack of health-related knowledge or skills may present obstacles to engaging in healthy behaviors, taking advantage of preventative services, and managing acute and chronic diseases [17]. Health literacy positively correlates with making better health-related decisions. Therefore, it is imperative that IP team members make health literacy a priority for patients and caregivers.

Health literacy can be accomplished through health classes, health groups, phone consultations, one-on-one meetings with health providers, and informational materials such as pamphlets. Whichever method is decided upon, giving attention to patient and caregiver learning styles can increase the effectiveness of health literacy. It is essential that both the patient and the caregiver absorb health-related information via their preferred learning style [18]. Learning styles include visual (watching the task performed), auditory (listening to an audio recording), kinesthetic (hands-on activities), and reading and writing. Teaching styles, which include explanation, verification, and demonstration, may also need to be tailored to the patient or the caregiver's intellectual and cognitive ability. Healthcare literacy can positively influence communication, patient compliance with treatment, and the patient's overall health status, all of which can result in cost savings to healthcare systems and improved patient-provider satisfaction [17]. Health literacy interventions have been linked to patients and caregivers being able to solve health problems more independently, thus resulting in fewer visits to emergency rooms [19].

Support Systems for Family Caregivers in Home Care Settings

According to a report by the American Association of Retired Persons (AARP) and the National Alliance of Caregiving (NAC), nearly 53 million (21.3% of US adults) serve as caregivers, providing $600 billion in unpaid care across the USA [20]. With this in mind, healthcare providers must show high regard for caregivers and be mindful of *caregiver burden*. Caregiver burden can be defined as the strain or load experienced by a person who is responsible for the care of another individual who is chronically ill, disabled, or older. This burden impacts both the caregiver and the patient and is reported to affect emotional wellness, physical health, social life and relationships, finances, and overall well-being [21]. To reduce the burden of care, external support systems and resources should be offered to assist the caregiver. Additionally, IP team members must avoid being rigid about care appointments or becoming impatient when providing instruction on caregiving tasks. Team members must avoid overwhelming caregivers with medical jargon, negative feedback, predictions about prognoses, or the cost of services [20]. Table 3.1 provides resources for family caregivers. These resources are supported federally, thus magnifying the importance of caregiver resources and supports. Federal subsidies also assure continuity of these essential resources as well as equity of access [22].

Table 3.1 Resources for family caregivers [22]

Resource	Description
National Family Caregiver Support Program (NFCSP)	Established in 2000 under Section 371 of the older Americans Act of 1965 (as amended, title IIIE), the NFCSP provides grants to states and territories to fund a range of supports that assist family and informal caregivers in caring for their loved ones at home for as long as possible
Eldercare locator	The eldercare locator is a public service of the US Administration on aging that helps caregivers locate resources for older adults in any US community
National Center on caregiving	The NCC serves as a central source of information on caregiving and long-term care issues for policymakers, service providers, media, funders, and family caregivers throughout the country
Caregiver Action Network (CAN)	The CAN is a nonprofit organization providing education, peer support, and resources to family caregivers nationwide free of charge
eXtension	eXtension is a website developed by the US Department of Agriculture (USDA) cooperative extension system that allows caregivers and advocates to access a wide range of information and materials related to disaster preparedness, housing, and nutrition

Characteristics and Responsibilities of Family Caregivers in the Home Care Milieu

The IP collaborative practice model places the position of the caregiver at its heart, connecting the domains of shared responsibility and values, communication, and teamwork. Assuming the role of a caregiver can be rewarding, but it can also be highly demanding. While the patient is the team captain, caregivers must be coaches and leaders. Active listening is essential to effective communication with the patient and the IP team. This skill helps the caregiver to understand the patient's wishes in order to accomplish care fruition [23]. Caregivers must possess the core values of altruism, caring, and compassion for the patient. They should also demonstrate respect for the patient and all members of the IP team. Caregivers should strive to understand the varied roles and functions of IP team members. They must be receptive to spending time with each provider, asking questions, and gaining knowledge about their responsibilities on the team. Communication with physicians, physician assistants, social workers, case managers, pharmacists, etc. is routine caregiver tasks [8].

Caregivers quickly learn to become care managers (e.g., retaining medical records in a designated location, maintaining a schedule of prescribed in-home activities, and keeping an up-to-date list of medications, appointments, and important contact numbers). Caregivers should keep at the ready a list of pertinent questions for IP team members so they can be easily accessed during provider visits. It is also recommended that caregivers maintain relevant notes pertaining to the patient's day-to-day progress and care. Caregivers can readily relay needed care information when notes are organized and dated. Additionally, caregivers must commit to being available to meet with team members as often as necessary. They may be required to participate in provider treatments, coordinate times for future home visits, and execute the patient's prescribed care program between visits [23].

Challenges Faced by Family Caregivers in Home Healthcare

Family caregivers must strive to balance their personal needs and the demands of caregiving. This can be done by soliciting support from other family members or the patient's significant others. Some caregivers tend to take on more responsibility than they can effectively handle. Thus, these caregivers benefit from delegating caregiving tasks to others. IP team members must actively listen to caregivers and anticipate their needs. They should support caregivers in their efforts to delegate caregiving tasks to others who are equally capable of caring for the patient. Caregivers need time for self-care, rest, and rejuvenation. Respite episodes are particularly important for employed caregivers and for those who are responsible for the care of minor children or other family members. Under these circumstances, the demands of caregiving can be challenging and overwhelming [24].

It is important that caregivers be supported in maintaining realistic goals (expectations) for themselves and their patients. Research findings have shown that caregiving has a significant impact on quality of life [8, 25–29]. Family caregivers may experience depression, anxiety, psychosomatic symptoms, restriction of roles and activities, strained marital relationships, and diminished physical health [30]. Other challenges encountered by caregivers may include the loss of identity or identity or role confusion. These experiences have the ability to impact patients and caregiver's quality of life.

Quality of Life and Wellness Considerations for Patients and Caregivers

Social isolation and loneliness are often experienced by older adults and those living with severe chronic illnesses. These individuals are often limited in their efforts to independently engage in activities of daily living [31]. While older adults do not have a higher rate of depression than the general population, this group is at a significantly higher risk for the development of depression [15]. Similarly, between 40% and 70% of caregivers exhibit symptoms of depression [32]. Research findings indicate that social isolation and loneliness are related to higher rates of major mental and physical illnesses (e.g., cardiovascular and cerebrovascular risks, depression, anxiety, increased risk of dementia), which poses possible health threats for both patient and caregiver [32]. Signs of depression may be manifested in the following manner [32]:

- Persistent sad, anxious, or "empty" mood.
- Feelings of hopelessness, guilt, worthlessness, or helplessness.

- Irritability, restlessness, or having trouble sitting still.
- Loss of interest in once pleasurable activities.
- Decreased energy or fatigue.
- Moving or talking more slowly.
- Difficulty concentrating, remembering, or making decisions.
- Difficulty sleeping, waking up too early in the morning, or oversleeping.
- Eating more or less than usual, usually with unplanned weight gain or loss.
- Thoughts of death or suicide or suicide attempts.

Loneliness and social isolation can also be experienced by caregivers when care demands hinder their ability to live a balanced life. Caregivers may have altered their formal routines, lifestyle, and social activities in order to focus on the patient, resulting in reduced time to connect with friends and social groups [32]. Regular communication among IP team members about the mood and affect of the patient and caregiver is important. When an IP team member suspects that the patient or caregiver is depressed or exhibiting severe anxiety, a referral should be made to the appropriate mental health authority. It is imperative to remember that the well-being of the caregiver directly impacts the well-being of the patient. The caregiver's ability or inability to adequately perform caregiving tasks can directly impact the quality of care rendered to the patient. Quality of care can significantly impact the patient care outcomes [33].

Client and Family Autonomy and Choice Making

To assure quality care and positive outcomes for home care patients, the basic principle of patient autonomy must be respected. Patient autonomy is formally defined as:

> The right of patients to make decisions about their medical care without their healthcare provider trying to influence the decision. Patient autonomy does allow for healthcare providers to educate the patient but does not allow the healthcare provider to make the decision for the patient [34].

Autonomy encompasses patients' freedoms to self-govern and make decisions that they believe are in their best interest. When providing healthcare in the home, IP team members must show their respect and appreciation for patient autonomy. This can be done by respecting requests and decisions relating to home modifications, adhering to the day and time of prescheduled home visits, and deciding what procedure or equipment is acceptable or necessary. The IP member can also demonstrate reverence for autonomy by respecting religious beliefs, religious holidays, and cultural and family norms. Desires to terminate services or change providers should also be respected. The necessity for patient autonomy is further emphasized during the establishment of the advanced directives, living will, medical power of attorney, and other estate planning activities. IP team members should not assert their opinions, beliefs, or biases when it comes to these very private matters.

Multicultural Considerations

When working in the home care milieu, it is imperative that providers understand the cultural perspectives of the patient and family. Understanding patient and family choices and lived experiences is important. Studies show that ethnic minority caregivers provide more caregiving support than their White counterparts [35]. Additionally, Asian American caregivers' use of professional support is significantly less than their White counterparts [36]. Research findings reveal that African American caregivers experience lower levels of caregiver burden and depression than White caregivers [36]. Hispanic and Asian American caregivers were more depressed than White caregivers [36]. The main reason for these divergences is that cultural perspectives differ across ethnic groups and impact caregivers' perceptions of the caregiving role, their utilization of support services, and clinical presentations and interactions [36]. While ethnicity is a dominant multicultural component, other factors such as sexual orientation, religion, gender, socioeconomic status, environment, and geographic location should be taken into consideration as well.

Home service providers, while not expected to know everything about a person's culture, are expected to acquire minimum competencies that would permit them to be mindful and respectful of patients and caregivers' cultural practices. Becoming culturally competent can promote insight into interventions that may or may not be desirable for the patient or family. Having this knowledge assures that interventions are tailored to fit the needs of patients and caregivers.

Chapter Summary

Now, more than ever, IP home healthcare teams are essential to providing high-quality and cost-effective services that improve health equity and healthcare outcomes. To that end, patient-centered care (coupled with IP team members' support and respect for family caregivers) is an essential function in achieving favorable patient outcomes. Caregiving is a rewarding yet tremendous responsibility. IP healthcare teams can reduce caregiver burden by being available and supportive of caregivers' needs. It is important to remember that the caregiver's ability or inability to adequately perform caregiving functions can directly impact care quality and patient health and wellness outcomes.

Case Study: Jeralean

The case study profiles the health status of Jeralean, a candidate for home healthcare services.

Jeralean is a 75-year-old African American woman with a right lower limb amputation distal to the knee, hypertension, type 2 diabetes, glaucoma, sleep apnea, constipation, painful neuropathy, and osteoarthritis. She complains of pain and stiffness in her fingers and wrists. She is not always compliant with her medications, frequently forgetting to take them. She reports having too many doctors and being on "too much medication." Jeralean was diagnosed with pneumonia twice in recent years. She presents with a poor appetite, weight loss (20 pounds in 6 months), anxiety, and sadness. Jeralean lost her husband of 45 years less than a year ago.

Jeralean spends a significant amount of time alone and does not desire to be around people. She spends most of her day sitting on the couch in her living room. She consumes large amounts of processed food that contains copious amounts of sodium, sugars, and fats which causes her glucose and blood pressure levels to be higher than normal. She reports "losing strength and energy." She sleeps very little at night and has difficulty falling asleep and remaining asleep.

Before her husband's death, the couple took daily walks, shared housekeeping tasks, and cooked most of their meals together. Her current medications include aspirin 81 mg daily, Lopressor 25 mg twice daily, metformin 500 mg twice daily, Lantus 7.5 units BID, NovoLog pen, Combigan 1 gtt os twice daily, Miralax 17 g/day, Neurontin 600 mg TID, Lyrica 100 mg TID, Tylenol #3-tab q 4 h as needed, and nortriptyline 50 mg daily. Jeralean has begun to have difficulty measuring her insulin correctly and giving her insulin shots during the day when her daughter is unavailable. She repeatedly has cuts on her left foot and her hands. She is often unaware of when the injuries occur and unable to gauge the severity of the injuries due to the already existing pain and numbness in the areas. Jeralean has been dropping things lately and has broken several glasses and plates because they slipped out of her hand.

Jeralean resides in a small rural southern county in the USA. Her 48-year-old daughter Alice resides with her and would love to see her remain at home for as long as possible. Alice states that until recently, her mother was meticulous about grooming and self-care and maintained a neat and orderly home. According to Alice, Jeralean has fallen three times recently: once in the bathroom, once in the kitchen, and once in the living room. She believes that her mother is experiencing some balance issues and vision loss. Jeralean no longer wears her prosthesis. She does not like for Alice to worry about her or to give her advice. She becomes angry when Alice attempts to provide physical assistance. While previously being quite social, Jeralean's current social interactions consist mostly of speaking with her siblings and staff at her doctors' offices.

Alice is an only child and works full-time as an accountant. Her place of employment is close to her mother's home. Therefore, she can "check on" Jeralean throughout the day on most days. Alice is in good health. She is divorced (for less than a year) and has no children. Her life priority at this point is to care for her mother. She worries about her once vibrant mother wasting away and giving up on life. Other than her daughter and sibling who reside out of state, Jeralean does not have a support system. At this time, she does not use a wheelchair or walker, or any other special or adaptive equipment. There are no handrails in the shower or anywhere else in the home. Currently, Jeralean travels over 60 miles to receive healthcare services.

Discussion Question

1. When considering the case of Jeralean, in what areas could she and her family be assisted with health literacy services and how might that service positively and/or negatively impact them?

Multiple Choice Questions

1. Which of the following best describes the term patient-centeredness?
   - (a) The interprofessional team approach to healthcare that places the patient at the center of care delivery and ensures that the patient's needs and values drive and guide clinical decisions.
   - (b) The interprofessional healthcare team meets with the patient and the caregiver in the patient's home to instruct the caregiver on techniques to provide quality care and assess the caregiver's ability to care for the patient.
   - (c) The team of healthcare providers meets with patients and families in a home environment to ensure that the caregiver is providing quality care to the patient.
   - (d) Interprofessional healthcare teams work collaboratively to decide what is best for the patient, based on their knowledge, expertise, and clinical judgment.
2. In 2010, the World Health Organization released a framework for interprofessional education and collaborative practice. Which of the following statements is *true* about the WHO framework for IPECP?
   - (a) The framework provides guidelines for healthcare professionals to learn from one another in academic settings.
   - (b) The framework provides guidelines for healthcare professionals to work collaboratively in clinical practice settings to develop and implement healthcare plans as a team.
   - (c) The framework promotes teams that are founded on mutual respect, shared values, and positive communication.

(d) All of these statements are true regarding the WHO framework for interprofessional education and collaborative practices.

3. Health literacy is best defined as

   (a) The degree to which individuals have the ability to find, understand, and use information and services to inform health-related decisions and actions for themselves and others
   (b) A patient who has achieved the highest level of difficulty in reading and understanding medical information related to his or her health condition
   (c) The capacity of a patient to determine the best course of care for themselves or their family members based on their reading comprehension
   (d) The ability of the person to gather health information from the Internet and social media sources to learn about health conditions

4. Which of the following *best* defines caregiver burden?

   (a) Caregiver burden is best defined as the strain or load of the person who is responsible for caring for a chronically ill, disabled, or older person that can impact the well-being and quality of life of both the patient and the caregiver.
   (b) Caregiver burden is best defined as the cross the caregiver must bear for the blessing they have received in life or the blessing they hope to receive in the future.
   (c) Caregiver burden refers to the cost of providing quality healthcare in the home environment related to the modifications and adaptations that the caregiver is required to make.
   (d) Caregiver burden refers to the physical lifting required by caregivers to assist patients who can't move from one surface to another or transition into different positions.

5. What is the primary role of the caregiver on the interprofessional healthcare team?

   (a) The primary role of the caregiver is to provide continuous support in a healing relationship for the patient whenever and wherever it is needed.
   (b) The primary role of the caregiver is to follow the instructions of the healthcare professionals and communicate them to the patient.
   (c) The primary role of the caregiver is to ensure that the healthcare providers show respect for the patient, keep their scheduled appointments, and report to the physician or home health agency about the quality of each healthcare provider.
   (d) All of the above.

6. Who are the caregivers?

   (a) Caregivers tend to be spouses, partners, family members, or neighbors who often assume the role without much training and preparation.
   (b) Caregivers are individuals from a home health agency whose sole purpose is to assist with daily activities and chores.

(c) Caregivers are typically the men of the family who can provide the most financial support for the patient.
(d) Caregivers are the individuals and family members who volunteer to care for patients because they have the most time and energy to support the patient.

References

1. Institute of Medicine. (2001). *Crossing the quality chasm: A new health system for the 21st century*. The National Academies Press. https://doi.org/10.17226/10027
2. Berwick, D. M., Nolan, T. W., & Whittington, J. (2008). The triple aim: Care, health, and cost. *Health Affairs, 27*(3), 759–769. https://doi.org/10.1377/hlthaff.27.3.759
3. World Health Organization. (2010, September 10). *Framework for Action on Interprofessional Education & Collaborative Practice*. World Health Organization. Retrieved May 7, 2023, from https://www.who.int/publications-detail- redirect/framework-for-action-on-interprofessional-education-collaborative-practice.
4. Interprofessional Education Collaborative Expert Panel. (2011). *Core competencies for interprofessional collaborative practice: Report of an expert panel*. Interprofessional Education Collaborative.
5. Interprofessional Education Collaborative. (2016). *Core competencies for interprofessional collaborative practice: 2016 update*. Interprofessional Education Collaborative.
6. Bodenheimer, T., & Sinsky, C. (2014). From triple to quadruple aim: Care of the patient requires care of the provider. *The Annals of Family Medicine, 12*(6), 573–576. https://doi.org/10.1370/afm.1713
7. Arnetz, B. B., Goetz, C. M., Arnetz, J. E., Sudan, S., vanSchagen, J., Piersma, K., & Reyelts, F. (2020). Enhancing healthcare efficiency to achieve the QUADRUPLE AIM: An exploratory study. *BMC Research Notes, 13*(1). https://doi.org/10.1186/s13104-020-05199-8
8. NASEM, Family Caregivers Alliance. (2016). *Caregiver statistics: Demographics*. https://www.caregiver.org/resource/caregiver-statistics-demographics/ I guess it was deleted. It was under challenges faced by caregivers–delete this.
9. National Academies of Sciences, Engineering, and Medicine. (2016). *Families caring for an aging America*. The National Academies Press. https://doi.org/10.17226/23606
10. Sinsky, C. A., Brown, R. L., Stillman, M. J., & Linzer, M. (2021). COVID-related stress and work intentions in a sample of US health care workers. *Mayo Clinic Proceedings: Innovations, Quality & Outcomes, 5*(6), 1165–1173. https://doi.org/10.1016/j.mayocpiqo.2021.08.007
11. Chandrasekhar, P., Moodley, S., & Jain, S. H. (2019). 5 Obstacles to home-based healthcare, and how to overcome them. *Harvard Business Review*. https://hbr.org/2019/10/5-obstacles-to-home-based-health-care-and-how-to-overcome-them#:~:text=These%20include%3A%20environmental%20hazards%20such,needs% 20of%20patients%20receiving%20home
12. Herbert, C., & Molinsky, J. (2019). What can be done to better support older adults to age successfully in their homes and communities? *Health Affairs, 38*(5), 860–864. https://doi.org/10.1377/hlthaff.2019.00203
13. Jayson, S. (2021, November 19). *How to make your home safe for aging parents*. AARP. Retrieved May 7, 2023, from https://www.aarp.org/caregiving/home-care/info- 2019/safety-tips.html.
14. Prado, P., Norman, R. S., Vasquez, L., Glassner, A., Osuoha, P., Meyer, K., Brackett, J. R., & White, C. L. (2022). An interprofessional skills workshop to teach family caregivers of people living with dementia to provide complex care. *Journal of Interprofessional Education & Practice, 26*. https://doi.org/10.1016/j.xjep.2021.100481
15. Centers for Disease Control & Prevention. (2022). *What is health literacy?* https://www.cdc.gov/healthliteracy/learn/index.html

16. Lopez, C., Kim, B., & Sacks, K. (2022). *Health literacy in the United States: Enhancing assessments and reducing disparities*. https://milkeninstitute.org/sites/default/files/2022-05/Health_Literacy_United_States_Final_Report.pdf
17. Phaneuf, M. (2013). *Teaching in caregiving*. http://www.prendresoin.org/wp-content/uploads/2013/11/Teaching-in-caregiving.pdf
18. Chesser, A., Woods, N., Smothers, K., & Rogers, N. (2015). Healthy literacy and older adults: A systematic review. *Gerontology & Geriatric Medicine, 2*, 1–13.
19. Liu, Z., Heffernan, C., & Tan, J. (2020). Caregiver burden: A concept analysis. *International Journal of Nursing Sciences, 7*(4), 438–445. https://doi.org/10.1016/j.ijnss.2020.07.012
20. Caldera, S., Houser, A., & Choula, R. (2023). *Valuing the invaluable 2023: Strengthening support for caregivers*. AARP Public Policy Institute. https://doi.org/10.26419/ppi.00082.008
21. Zolbin, M., Huvila, I., & Nikou, S. (2022). Health literacy, health literacy interventions and decision making: A systematic literature review. *Journal of Documentation, 78*(7), 405–428.
22. USDHHS. (2023).
23. Underwood, A., Watson, S., & Booth, B. (2015). *Caregiver's handbook: A guide to caring for the ill, elderly, or disabled-and yourself.* Harvard Medical School.
24. Akçoban, S., & Eskimez, Z. (2023). Homecare patients' quality of life and the burden of family caregivers: A descriptive cross-sectional study. *Home Health Care Services Quarterly*, 1–14. https://doi.org/10.1080/01621424.2023.2177224
25. Sales, E. (1991). Psychosocial impact of the phase of cancer on the family. *Journal of Psychosocial Oncology, 9*, 1–9.
26. Ell, K., Nishimoto, R., Mantell, J., & Hamovitch, M. (1988). Longitudinal analysis of psychosocial adaptation among family members of patients with cancer. *Journal of Psychosomatic Research, 32*, 429–438.
27. Johnson, J. (1988). Cancer. *Recent Result Cancer Research, 108*, 306–310.
28. Pederson, L. M., & Valanis, B. G. (1988). The effects of breast cancer on the family. *Journal Psychosocial Oncology, 6*, 95–118.
29. Toseland, R. W., Blanchard, C. G., & McCallion, P. (1998). A problem-solving intervention for caregivers of cancer patients. *Social Science Medicine, 40*, 517–528.
30. Committee on Family Caregiving for Older Adults; Board on Health Care Services; Health and Medicine Division; National Academies of Sciences, Engineering, and Medicine; Schulz R., Eden, J. editors. Families Caring for an Aging America. Washington (DC). National Academies Press (US); 2016 Nov 8. 3, Family Caregiving Roles and Impacts.
31. Townsend, E. (2020). *Home health care can help seniors with loneliness and social isolation*. Retrieved from https://www.heartsforhospiceandhomehealth.com/home- health-care-can-help-seniors-with-loneliness-and-social-isolation/
32. Wellness Everyday. (2023). *Caregiver stress*. Retrieved from https://www.wellnesseveryday.org/caregiver-loneliness
33. Alonazi, W., & Thomas, S. (2014). Quality of care and quality of life: Convergence or divergence? *Health Service Insights., 10*(7), 1–12.
34. Marks, J. (2021). *Medical definition of patient autonomy*. MedicineNet. https://www.medicinenet.com/patient_autonomy/definition.htm
35. McCann, J., Hebert, L., Beckett, M., Scherr, P., & Evans, D. (2000). Comparison of informal caregiving by black and white older adults in a community population. *Journal of the American Geriatrics Society, 48*, 1612–1617.
36. American Psychological Association. (2011). *Cultural diversity and caregiving*. American Psychological Association.

Chapter 4
Medical Social Work and Case Management

Tracy Pressley, Shanae Shaw, and Tabitha Brookins

Learning Objectives

1. Understand medical social workers' roles in providing care to older patients in diverse clinical settings.
2. Recognize the advantages and disadvantages of providing care in home care or natural settings.
3. Understand the person-in-environment approach.
4. Articulate safety and crisis planning considerations for older patients and their families.
5. Identify common workplace hazards.
6. Describe strategies social workers and other home care workers can use to protect themselves from workplace violence.
7. Describe strategies employers can use to protect home care staff from workplace violence.

Introduction

In hospitals and other healthcare clinical settings, medical social workers are acknowledged as being on the front line of providing services to patients and their families. Their functions are relative to the hospital system, the environment, the family system, and the community and social systems. In clinical settings, medical social workers provide support, such as helping to explain diagnoses, providing treatment options, and identifying and meeting the needs of patients after being discharged. Medical social workers assist patients and families in accessing community care and treatment resources, such as elder care services, government

Supplementary Information The online version contains supplementary material available at https://doi.org/10.1007/978-3-031-40889-2_4.

T. Pressley (✉) · S. Shaw · T. Brookins
Department of Social Work, College of Liberal Arts and Social Sciences, Alabama State University, Montgomery, AL, USA
e-mail: tpressley@alasu.edu; sshaw@alasu.edu; tbrookins@alasu.edu

D. H. Stapleton, S. Bossie (eds.), *Home Care for Older Adults Using Interprofessional Teams*, https://doi.org/10.1007/978-3-031-40889-2_4

programs, meal delivery services, or pharmacy assistance programs [1]. Central to the functions of the medical social worker are case management tasks. Case management is not a profession unto itself but a profession of cross-disciplinary practice from nursing to social work. Case management is a "professional and collaborative process that assesses, plans, implements, coordinates, monitors, and evaluates the options and services required to meet an individual's health needs." [2] According to the Commission for Case Manager Certification, the case management process is guided by nine interactive steps: (1) screening, (2) assessing, (3) stratifying risk, (4) planning, (5) implementation, (6) care coordination, (7) follow-up, (8) transitional care and communicating post-transition, and (9) evaluating [2]. Case managers help patients coordinate and navigate their healthcare journey in a cost-effective manner.

Refer to Table 4.1 for a complete list of the case management functions of medical social workers in the healthcare setting. These are standard social work practices

Table 4.1 Case management functions of medical social workers

Assess patient's priorities, strengths, and challenges	Understand common ethical and legal issues in social work practice
Monitor service delivery	Use of the strength's perspective and biopsychosocial-spiritual assessment
Ensure patient has the requisite information to provide informed consent in all aspects of the case management process	Engage the patient and family in all aspects of social work intervention
	Discharge and transition planning
	Advance care planning
	Hospice and end-of-life care
	Identification of elder or vulnerable adult abuse, trauma, neglect, and exploitation
Make the necessary transfer or referral if the patient still needs such a service to ensure continuity of care	Facilitate benefits and resource acquisition to assist patients and families, including understanding related policies, eligibility requirements, and financial and legal issues
Discharge planning	
Resource management	Advocate with other members of the interprofessional team and within the healthcare institution to promote patients' and families' decision-making and quality of life
	Provide patient and family interprofessional and community education
Coordinate care among all team members	Knowledgeable of family system issues, including the impact of healthcare concerns, illness, and disease on family relationships, life cycles, and caregiving roles and support needs
Ensure patient knowledge and compliance with treatment	
Coordinate care team meetings	Utilization management
Verify benefits and authorization of services	
Serve as a liaison between providers and the insurance company	
Monitor for compliance with the treatment or care plan	
Ensure appropriate level of care and care setting	
Provide education about healthcare benefits	

[3–5]. As the table indicates, these roles and responsibilities are vast. They are pivotal in most phases of patient care (e.g., assessment; risk identification; care plan development, implementation, and monitoring; patient education; care coordinating, community linkage, and resource development; advocacy and discharge planning).

Additionally, medical social workers must demonstrate proficiency in the following areas:

Crisis Management

Medical social workers assist patients who experience or have unplanned crises, often with devastating results. The social worker must be ready to help the patient and family cope with the aftermath of the crisis.

Psychosocial Assessment and Psychological Review

Medical social workers perform psychosocial assessments on patients and family members to identify needs and concerns that could exacerbate the patients' health conditions. The psychosocial assessment comprises evaluating psychological and physical health and the degree to which external and internal factors (e.g., financial hardship, biological and physiological changes, family conflict, cultural considerations) influence patient outcomes. After completing the assessment, medical social workers communicate with team members, such as nurses, physicians, physical therapists, occupational therapists, dietitians, and medical assistants, about their findings and investigate ways to provide the best possible patient care. Psychosocial assessment and reviews of psychological evaluations are conducted for the purpose of treatment planning and intervention implementation. This diagnostic information facilitates an understanding of the patient, the patient's social environment, and the integration of the patient's needs with the social environment.

Service and Intervention Planning

It is critical that medical social workers develop and implement a comprehensive and goal-directed treatment or care plan that comprises appropriate goals, interventions, strategies, and supports.

Counseling and Education

An essential role in medical social work is the provision of education about diagnoses and medical conditions. Emotional support may include psychotherapy, cognitive behavioral therapy, mindfulness-based stress reduction, and solution-focused therapy. Educating geriatric patients and their families post-discharge about resources within the community is also a vital function.

Care Coordination

Care coordination is defined as the effective organization and delivery of medical care to patients. Medical social workers must ensure that patients' medical, emotional, family, and social concerns are incorporated into their treatment (care) plan and that patients receive holistic and compassionate care.

Natural Clinical Environment Versus Other Clinical Settings

Many older patients struggle with the decision to either remain at home or move to an alternative care location. To make a well-informed decision, family, caregivers, and healthcare professionals must understand the benefits and harms of the various care options [6]. Standard long-term care options include home care and institutional care [7]. Home care typically includes independent living or living at home with support and modifications in place to enhance health and independence. Institutional care options typically refer to nursing home care or skilled nursing facilities. Older patients and their caregivers have identified moving from home to an alternative care option as one of their most challenging decisions [8, 9]. However, this decision is complicated by the evolving contextual factors related to the care situation, such as the patient's health status, the characteristics of the caregivers, and the physical environment [8].

Benefits and Limitations of Providing Care in the Skilled Nursing or Hospital Setting

The most significant benefit of being cared for in a skilled nursing or hospital setting is that skilled medical professionals are readily available, and timely treatment can be administered if health begins to deteriorate. Assistance is available for cleaning, walking, bathing, or dressing, and nutritious meals are consistently offered. However, these settings are more restrictive care environments. They are primarily for patients who require higher levels of monitoring following an illness, medical procedure, or emergency. Once their health improves, these patients are considered for home care. Skilled nursing facilities are often recommended for patients with multimorbidity or those with Alzheimer's or dementia, particularly if they are prone to wandering or aggression. Skilled nursing facilities are staffed with a variety of professionals who provide medical and nonmedical care around the clock. Hospitals and skilled nursing facilities have specific or limited visiting hours for family and friends. Many long-term care settings face challenges such as staff turnover, insufficient staff training, and inadequate time for patient and family consultations. All of these factors can adversely impact patient outcomes. Additionally, hospitals and skilled nursing facilities can be expensive, especially those of high quality. Today's demographics are shifting toward an aging population with complex healthcare needs that present many healthcare challenges in providing long-term care [10].

Benefits and Limitations of Providing Care in the National Clinical Environment

As the number and proportion of older adults in the population continues to increase, so does the demand for in-home geriatric services. Research shows that a large proportion of older adults prefer to remain in their own homes. A universal desire to age in place is the preference of many because it affords the opportunity to stay at home where the environment is familiar, and neighbors can be relied on for assistance and socializing. Aging-at-home affords the patient with a greater sense of personal control. The location of care (LOC) for older adults is an increasingly important societal concern [11].

There is increasing pressure to provide health and social care at home to reduce costs relative to institutional care [12–14]. A primary advantage of home-based services is that social workers have the opportunity to observe clients in their natural environments. Many seniors are more relaxed in their own space. Home-based services are also convenient for patients who cannot drive or travel to a clinical office setting. One challenge to providing care in the home setting pertains to the maintenance of professional boundaries. Typically, working in an office-based or inpatient setting minimizes the likelihood of boundary confusion. Visits are structured and occur in professional and confidential settings. In contrast, home-based services are less formal and structured and occur in the patient's personal space. Thus, social workers may be inclined to become more casual in their duties and relationships with patients and family members. Confidentiality is another challenge to providing care in the home setting. Protecting sensitive and confidential information may be difficult despite a social worker's best efforts. Depending on the home's configuration, it may be taxing to find a private space to talk or to conduct an assessment. The only quiet or private space may be the patient's bedroom or garage. Moreover, the presence of family and significant others in the home setting can distract both provider and patient from focusing on vital aspects of care.

The Person-in-Environment Approach

The practice of social work is guided by the person-in-environment, or "PIE," theoretical framework. Under this framework, social workers describe how people are influenced by their environment. The PIE approach focuses on the importance of understanding patients and their behavior relative to their environment. Environment and experiences shape how their patients view the world, how they think, and why they respond the way they do. This model suggests that the environment continuously changes as the older person takes from it what is needed, controls what can be modified, and adapts to conditions that cannot be changed. Adaptation implies a dual process in which the patient adjusts to characteristics of the social and physical environments.

Different system levels within the PIE approach are micro, mezzo, and macro, which help to dictate the type of support needed.

Microlevel: This comprises individual needs and involves direct interactions with the patient. This is the most common type of social work. This is a level that explores aspects related to biology, psychological needs, social (peer) and interpersonal (family) relationships or supports, and spiritual beliefs.

Jeralean's microlevel: Physical health issues related to 75-year-old Jeralean have been reported along with noncompliance with her medication; difficulty falling asleep; poor appetite, anxiety, and sadness; and no memory of when her injuries occur. The daughter's reports indicate a need for support from the environment so the person (her mother) can remain in her home. This support from the environment can be in-home supportive services or in-home health to assist her mother in staying at home. Jeralean is not only experiencing biological changes (inability to sleep and a decline in memory), but psychological and social changes have occurred due to significant life events such as losing her husband and physical changes. No spiritual beliefs were reported in the vignette but would need to be explored when meeting with Jeralean.

- *Mezzo-Level:* This comprises connections or interactions with small groups, such as family, churches, neighborhoods, community organizations, and peers.

Jeralean's mezzo-level: The worker needs to determine how her relationship and interaction with various groups impact her family, peers, possible spiritual affiliation or church, and any other community or organization she identifies being connected with.

- *Macro-Level:* This comprises connections to systemic issues within a large system, such as laws and legislation, policy, healthcare systems, and international associations. This level explores ethical frameworks, historical impacts on group experiences, and how discrimination and prejudice can impact marginalized populations such as older adults.

Jeralean's macro-level: Age policies, mental health policies, healthcare systems, cultural and historical impacts of group experience, and possible prejudice and discrimination should be examined.

- It is essential to examine each level (micro, mezzo, and macro) and explore the interconnectedness and interactions between what information is presented on each level and the impact it has on patients' function and development within their environment.

Accentuating Traditional Assessment Procedures and Evaluating Patient Needs

Assessment "aims to identify and explain the nature of a problem, to appraise it within and evaluate it within a framework of a specific element, and to use that appraisal as a guide to action" [15]. The primary objective of a medical social work assessment is to develop an acceptable intervention plan with reasonably attainable treatment goals [16]. An assessment is a diagnostic procedure used to examine varied patient-specific issues for the purpose of selecting appropriate interventions or treatment modalities. The patient and family assessment results are used to match a patient with needed services and care along a continuum of care [17]. Assessing activities of daily living (ADLs) and instrumental activities of daily living (IADLs) can help families determine the best types of support and care options. Two popular assessments of ADLs include KATZ Index of Independence in Activities of Daily Living [18–20] and Instrumental Activities of Daily Living Scale [21]. Psychosocial assessments (previously discussed) are conducted to determine patients' needs and to identify any mental or emotional distress that could exacerbate their medical condition.

Other assessment tools used by medical social workers include the Diagnostic and Statistical Manual (DSM) [22], Beck Depression Inventory [23], or the Mini-Mental Status Exam (MMS) [24]. As members of interprofessional teams, social workers advocate for the use of appropriate assessments with older patients who experience challenges due to multiple social determinants of health (SDOH) in the community [25]. As "context specialists," social workers strive to understand the needs of older adults receiving in-home services by considering those factors that impact their lives and well-being. Because social work practice is informed by the PIE perspective, social workers, in collaboration with older adult patients, can examine their needs and environment in order to determine the most appropriate interventions. Aligned with this perspective, social workers' assessments are influenced by the biopsychosocial approach [26].

As people age, the possibility of living with two or more chronic illnesses (multimorbidity) may increase. Health outcomes are diminished when the physical environment, social and cultural determinants, healthcare, and behavioral risk factors interact unfavorably. Comprehensive assessments are needed to develop effective plans to address issues relating to intersectionality. Such assessments should be championed by all interprofessional team members.

Safety Considerations, Crisis Planning, Emergency Preparedness

Older patients are most vulnerable to falls because with aging, reaction time and ability starts to wane. The time required to recover is also longer due to the slow recovery process [27]. Poor lighting, slippery floors, clutter, unsecured mats, stair climbing, and standing on stools can place the patient at risk for a fall. The number of falls increases with age. It is estimated that 28–35% of people aged 65 and above and 32–34% of people aged 70 years fall each year [28–30]. It is essential to note that opioids and benzodiazepines (BZD) are commonly prescribed medications that contribute to falls in older adults. Identifying the prevalence of falls and associated factors contributing to them will aid in instituting preventative measures. Below is a complete list of (evidence-based) elder fall risk tools that social workers and others can utilize to assess the likelihood of a patient falling.

- Berg Balance Scale
- Conley Fall Risk Assessment
- Downtown Fall Risk Assessment
- Elderly Fall Screening
- Elderly Mobility Scale
- Fall Risk Assessment
- Hendrich Fall Risk Assessment
- Innes Fall Risk Assessment
- Johns Hopkins Fall Risk Assessment
- Morse Fall Risk Assessment
- Schmid Fall Risk Assessment
- St. Thomas Risk Assessment Tool (STRATIFY)
- Timed Up and Go Test
- Tinetti Balance Scale

Violence in the Home Care Setting

Another safety consideration is workplace violence. Medical social workers must acknowledge the possibility of violence occurring in the home setting. They must be cognizant of the patient's community, know how to avoid violent situations, and be aware of organizational policies and procedures pertaining to violence de-escalation and avoidance. Home care workers are susceptible to verbal abuse, aggression, threats, and sexual harassment. Thus, active measures should be taken to prevent, identify, and eliminate factors impacting safety. This is an area where interprofessional teaming and collaboration can be of great benefit.

Assessing threats to safety is a continuous function. Organizations should offer avoidance training and verbal and violence de-escalation training during orientation and at least once annually. The skills introduced require continuous attention and practice. During home visits, social workers must remain alert to their surroundings and to signs of potential violence demonstrated by the patient or others in the home setting.

Home Care Safety

Home care safety can be divided into three categories: workers' responsibility to protect their own safety, the agency or organization's responsibility to train workers and provide safe practice in the workplace, and patients' and families' responsibility to promote the safety of the interprofessional team member. In the following paragraphs, we will provide specifics pertaining to each of the three categories.

In-Home Safety Checklist (for Use with Patients) As physical and cognitive capacities change, it may become more challenging for some older individuals to safely navigate their home environments. Thus, it is essential for social workers to evaluate the home for safety hazards that might impede a patient's ability to carry out necessary activities of daily living. The CDC provides examples of home areas that should be promptly assessed [31]. Table 4.2 depicts some guiding questions that can be useful in assessing home safety. These questions are a checklist of sorts. Any "yes" response requires a deliberate action such as the ones provided in Table 4.2. Thousands of falls occur annually within the home setting. Unfortunately, for older persons, these falls often result in serious injury or death. Thus, assisting patients and families in maintaining a hazard-free living space is important.

Ensuring Employee Safety Organizations can use a checklist from the 2010 National Institute for Occupational Safety and Health (NIOSH) to promote employee safety in the home care setting. The checklist can be found in *The Hazard Review: Occupational Hazards in Home Health Care*. Below are some pertinent questions from the checklist for organizations to consider. The full checklist can be downloaded from the NIOSH website [32].

Floors: Look at the floor in each room
Q: When you walk through a room do you have to walk around furniture? • Ask someone to move the furniture so your path is clear. **Q: Do you have throw-rugs on the floor?** • Remove the rugs or use a double-sided tape or a non-slip backing so the rugs don't slip **Q: Are there papers, books, towels, blankets, or other objects on the floor?** • Pick up things that are on the floor. Always keep objects off the floor.
Stairs and steps: Look at the stairs you use both and outside your home
Q: Are there papers, shoes, books, or other objects on the stairs? • Pick up things on the stairs. Always keep objects off the stairs. **Q: Are some steps broken or uneven** • Fix loose or uneven steps. **Q: Do you have only one light switch for your stairs (only at the top or bottom of the stairs)?** • Have an electrician put in a light switch at the top and bottom of the stairs. You can get light switches that glow. **Q: Are the handrails on the stairs loose or broken? Is there a handrail on only one side of the stairs?** • Fix loose handrails or put in new ones. Make sure handrails are on both sides of the stairs and are the length of the stairs

Table 4.2 Questions to ask when assessing home safety [31]

Kitchen: Look at your kitchen and eating area
Q: Are the things you often use on high shelves? • Keep things used often on lower shelves **Q: Is your step stool sturdy?** • If you must use a step stool get one with a bar to hold on to. Never use a chair as a step stool.
Bedrooms: Look at all your bedrooms
Q: Is the light near the bed hard to reach? • Place the lamp close to the bed where it's easy to reach. **Q: Is the path from your bed to the bathroom dark?** • Put a nightlight so you can see where you walk.
Bathrooms: Look at all your bathrooms
Q: Is the tub or shower floor slippery? • Put non-slip rubber mat or self-stick strips on floor of tub or shower **Q: Do you need support when you get in and out of the tub or from the toilet?** • Have grab bars put next to and inside the tub and next to the toilet.

Tab. 4.2 (continued)

- Are workers taught how to identify verbal abuse and what to do about it?
- Does an active safety program exist with a safety manager and safety committee that comprises employees from across the organization?
- Does annual training review or identify new safety issues from the previous year?
- Does an animal-control policy exist requiring animals to be restrained during home visits?

Patient and Family Responsibilities Patients and their families have a responsibility to create safe environments for home care personnel. They should be provided with documentation from the organization that details their responsibilities as recipients of home care services. Examples of patient responsibilities comprise the following:

- Agreeing and adhering to the worker's safety information and organizational policies
- Informing the home care worker of potential hazards, such as a guard dog, during the initial call to schedule a home visit
- Agreeing to restrain pets during visits
- Removing tripping hazards in the home or being willing to remove hazards during the visit
- Providing an escort (patient, family member, or friend) to walk home care personnel to their car in a high-crime neighborhood
- Refraining from shouting or swearing at home care personnel
- Refraining from inappropriately touching the home care personnel
- Limiting violent family members' access during the home visit

Emergency Preparedness

In 2017, the Centers for Medicare and Medicaid Services (CMS) established national emergency requirements for all participating organizations, including hospitals, home health agencies, and hospices. Organizations must have a functional emergency preparedness program that describes their comprehensive approach to meeting the health, safety, and security needs of the care organization, its staff, and the patient population. Federal, state, and local governments have created universal emergency and disaster planning standards for healthcare organizations. Government units such as Homeland Security, the Federal Emergency Management Agency, and the Centers for Disease Control have developed these standards in concert with the state and county public health or health and human service units.

Emergency Preparedness: Healthcare Organizations

Most governments expect healthcare organizations to adopt and implement an emergency planning protocol in order to maximize resources in the event of a disaster or emergency. The protocol should be integrated into broader or national emergency preparedness requirements. Box 4.1 provides a basic protocol that organizations can employ to examine hazards and disasters that have the potential to disrupt service delivery and impact the safety and well-being of all stakeholders.

Box 4.1 Protocol for Examining Hazards and Disaster

1. Review CMS national emergency requirements.
2. Identify potentially hazardous or disastrous events for your organization and practice settings.
3. Evaluate each event for probability (values should range from 1-*low* to 5-*high*).
4. Evaluate each event for vulnerability (values should range from 1-*low* to 5-*high*).
5. Evaluate each event for preparedness (values should range from 1-*low* to 5-*high*).
6. When evaluating probability, consider the frequency and likelihood an event may occur.
7. When evaluating vulnerability, consider the degree with which the organization will be impacted (e.g., infrastructure damage, loss of life, service disruption, communication systems).
8. When evaluating preparedness, consider elements, such as the strength of your current preparedness plans and the organization's previous experience with the hazardous or disastrous event.
9. Those rated as *moderate* (a value of 3) or *high* (a value of 5) require immediate and deliberate action in order to increase emergency readiness and preparedness.
10. Identify current needs and deficiencies that must be addressed in order to maximize emergency readiness and preparedness.
11. Identify available resources that can be used during an emergency situation.
12. Determine which values represent an acceptable risk level and which values require additional planning and preparation.
13. All organizational members shall be involved in identifying and formulating solutions to potentially hazardous or disastrous events within the organization and practice settings.

Emergency Preparedness: The Patient and Family

Figure 4.1 addresses emergency preparedness for individuals with special needs relating to verbal communication, hearing, blindness or low vision, and mobility. Many patients who are older experience these challenges. These medical conditions may be acquired or congenital. Congenital disabilities are conditions that have been present since birth. The information depicted in Fig. 4.1 is a valuable resource for emergency planning and should be discussed with patients and families.

Speech or communication Issues

If you use a laptop computer for communication, consider getting a power converter that plugs into the cigarette lighter

Hearing Issues

Have a pre-printed copy of key phrase messages handy, such as "I use American Sign Language (ASL)," I do not write or read English well, and "If you make announcements, I will need to have them written simply or signed."

Consider getting a weather radio with a visual/text display that warns of the weather emergencies.

Vision Issues

Mark your disaster supplies with fluorescent tape, large print, or Braille

Have high-powered flashlights with wide beams and extra batteries

Place security lights in each room to light paths of travel.

Assistive Device Users

Label equipment with simple instruction cards on how to operate it (for example, how to "free wheel" or "disengage the gears" of your power wheelchair) Attach the cards to your equipment.

If you use a cane, keep extras in strategic, consistent, and secure locations to help you maneuver around obstacles and hazards.

Keep a spare cane in your emergency kit.

Know what your options are if you are not able to evacuate with your assistive device.

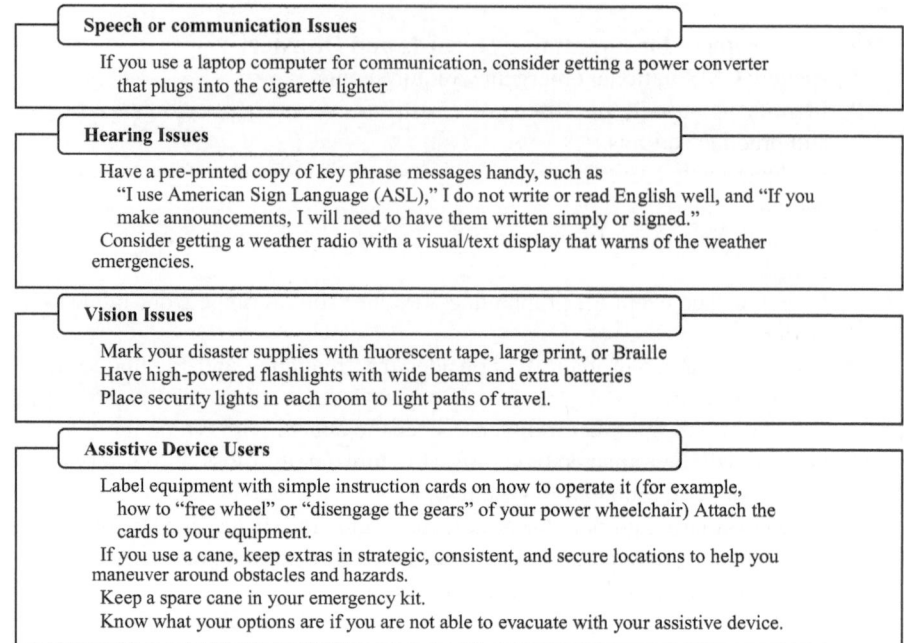

Fig. 4.1 Emergency preparedness for people with special needs

Telehealth

There are many benefits of telehealth services. In addition to serving as an ideal method for the provision of care during a global pandemic, telehealth also benefits patients who reside in rural communities. Through telehealth services, individuals in rural communities and those with mobility limitations have an opportunity to receive quality healthcare services. From a patient-centered perspective, telehealth services are often considered comfortable and convenient, specifically for patients who live far away from the providing agency and do not have access to reliable transportation [33, 34].

While the benefits of telehealth services have a positive impact on health outcomes for those who reside in rural communities. There are also several drawbacks to telehealth service use. One concern is related to the use of technology. Because technological systems are always evolving, there is a concern that the focus of telehealth may shift from a service that is patient-centered to one that revolves around securing the newest piece of technology. An additional concern about telehealth relates to technology literacy. E-health literacy refers to an individual's ability to "seek, find, understand, and appraise health information from electronic sources and apply the knowledge gained to addressing and solving a health problem" [35]. In a study that examined the use of eHealth literacy among older adults (aged 55 and older) who were patients in clinics serving low-income populations, there was lower general Internet use among older adults with increasing age, lower educational attainment, and minority ethnic status [36]. In a similar study exploring the perceived ease of use and feasibility of mobile health applications, study results highlighted that smartphone technology and other health-related computer technologies were not preferred by older adult study participants [37].

Preparing for a Telehealth Appointment

There are several steps that a medical social worker must take before scheduling and participating in a telehealth appointment with a patient. This preparation can be conducted in steps, which are found below. However, depending on the patient's previous experience with telehealth appointments, some steps below may be skipped. For example, if the patient has already met with the social worker via electronic communication, the social worker might forgo the process of assisting the patient with the setup of new Internet coverage.

Step 1: Consider the Patient's Interest

During the process of scheduling an appointment with a patient, the medical social worker needs to consider the patient's interest in a telehealth format. If the patient is not open to participating via telehealth, the social worker might explore both formal and informal resources to assist the patient with participating in a face-to-face appointment. The social worker should always consider agency policies and practices when discussing service options with a patient.

Step 2: Obtain Informed Consent

In most cases, the medical social worker will be required to obtain informed consent from the patient before engaging in telehealth communication. Concerning telehealth services, an informed consent document should make the patient aware of expectations and responsibilities during the appointment, risks and benefits of participation in telehealth services, and alternative methods to providing the service. The informed consent document should be signed by the patient and returned to the social worker or agency before the appointment.

Step 3: Ensure Access to Internet or Phone Service

Once a patient has expressed interest in receiving telehealth services, the medical social worker must then ensure that the patient has the proper equipment to participate in the appointment. In most cases, the proper equipment will include a working telephone or in-home Internet service. If the appointment is taking place through the use of a videoconferencing platform, the social worker will need to ensure that the patient has access to a computer or laptop on the date and time of the appointment. If a patient does not have access to in-home Internet service, the social worker should seek to secure community resources or programs that can establish this service in the patient's home. Social workers must also acknowledge and address any accessibility needs which may include providing auxiliary aids and services.

Step 4: Prepare for the Appointment

To ensure privacy, the patient and social worker need to arrange an appointment in a private space. The social worker should share this requirement with the patient immediately following the scheduling of the appointment. This allows time for the patient to make the needed arrangements. Patients should not participate in telehealth communication in public or semipublic spaces [38]. Additional activities to prepare for a telehealth appointment include testing Internet strength and ensuring proper operation of audio or visual platforms. Testing a patient's Internet strength or deciding which room of the home offers the best Internet connection is an important step in the telehealth service process. These steps ensure the efficacy and efficiency of the appointment. Similarly, social workers must have a thorough understanding of their agency's telehealth software. Social workers should share with the patient the course of action should technical glitches occur during the appointment. Social workers should consult agency policies and procedures when preparing patients for such circumstances.

Interprofessional Collaboration

The primary goal of an interprofessional team is to apply multiple perspectives in the treatment of patients to ensure their medical and emotional needs are met [39]. It is essential for social workers to not only ensure that interprofessional collaboration is grounded in the person-in-environment approach but to also make sure that interprofessional team members understand the benefits of the person-in-environment approach. This approach not only increases the "range of available interventions, with options to intervene directly with the individual or into other aspects of the environment, or both" [40]. The identification of this range of interventions at both the individual and community levels provides an increased opportunity for interprofessional teams to not only address the client's primary concern but to also support the sustainment of the patient's environment. The incorporation of an interprofessional healthcare model increases staff satisfaction and retention and greater perceptions of empowerment and recognition [41, 42]. Interprofessional collaboration can lead to "improved communication among providers, which further ensures that patients receive the best possible care" [43]. An effective way to improve health outcomes for older adults with complex medical and social needs is to implement interprofessional collaboration with allied and healthcare professionals [44–47]. Members of interprofessional teams often have ties to the community being served and provide interventions in the homes of patients with complex medical issues. They are often found to be effective at addressing the social determinants of health that lead to poor clinical outcomes. Through collaborative practice, interprofessional teams are able to address a myriad of patient factors by incorporating culturally and linguistically competent interventions.

Coordinating Medical Services and Referrals

A referral of services is the request or demand for additional services to meet a patient's needs [48]. The initiation of a referral of services takes place when a patient's current agency or organization does not provide a specific service or skill set that will assist the patient in meeting personal, medical, psychological, or social goals. For example, a social worker provides psychosocial services to a 67-year-old patient to assist in the readjustment to the home setting. While conducting the initial assessment, the social worker discovers that the patient's spouse passed away 2 months prior. The social worker may consider referring the patient to a local agency that provides grief counseling, should further assessment warrant this type of intervention. Often a referral is informed by interprofessional collaboration. Social workers making referrals should strive to stay abreast of their patients' progress and levels of satisfaction.

Resolving Interprofessional Conflict and Disagreement Among IP Team Members

Given the varying roles, training, perspectives, and experiences of the various members of the interprofessional team, it should not be a surprise that such diversity coupled with the desire to help a patient sometimes results in disagreement or conflict between team members or among the team as a whole. When this happens, social workers can play an essential role in assisting the team in resolving conflict. Due to the nature of social work and the interpersonal and communication skills that social workers must possess in order to identify both the needs of patients and corresponding resources, social workers are adept at conflict management and resolution.

There are two sources of conflict, substantive conflict and emotional conflict [49]. Substantive conflict refers to conflict related to the scope of practice and differing philosophical perspectives regarding patient care [49]. On the other hand, emotional conflicts reflect conflicting personality differences among interprofessional teams [49]. Regardless of the type of conflict, interprofessional team members need to identify the source of the conflict and work to resolve it promptly. Failure to resolve conflict has the potential to negatively affect patient outcomes. In addition to impacting the care environment, the unresolved conflict also has the potential to take team members' attention away from the patient which certainly influences the performance of the interprofessional team [50].

Regardless of the nature of the practice conflict, evidence-informed interventions should take precedence when determining how to proceed in helping a patient. Amid conflict, interprofessional team members must be open to listening to the rationale of other team members, discussing their personal feelings or thoughts about a particular intervention, and reflecting on all team members' perspectives [51]. If interprofessional collaboration emphasizes putting the patient first, supporting autonomy and self-determination, and implementing least restrictive intervention options, then care providers can decrease the chances of interprofessional conflict interfering with patient care and outcomes.

Chapter Summary

This chapter highlighted the integral role of medical social workers in diverse care settings as well as the benefits and limitations of each setting. It highlighted the significance of case management which is a vital medical social work function. This chapter also discussed safety considerations, from fall risks and home hazards to workplace violence and emergency preparedness. Interprofessional collaboration is central to the provision of patient-centered and holistic care. This type of approach to service provision can have a positive impact on not only patient outcomes but the overall culture of the work environment for interprofessional team members. Telehealth services provide an opportunity for social workers to provide services to patients who are unable to participate in a face-to-face appointment due to distance, transportation, or health condition. Social workers must take the necessary steps to ensure the privacy, comfortability, and overall effectiveness of a telehealth appointment. The practice of social work is guided by the person-in-environment theoretical framework which describes how people are influenced by their environment.

Discussion Questions

1. Describe the risk and benefits of providing home care services to older clients and patients?
2. Why is it important that families have an emergency preparedness plan?

Assignment

Imagine Jeralean residing in your community. Search the Internet and locate at least five available home care facilities to assist Jeralean in staying in her home. Also, explain how these facilities are similar or different from each other.

Assignment: "Make a Plan" Activity

1. Medical social workers are critical in assisting seniors and their caregivers in the disaster preparedness and response plan. Use the provided emergency preparedness checklist to create your emergency plan.

   Completing this "make a plan" activity will help you know what to do in an emergency. It will take you about 20 min to make your plan. Your family may not be together when an emergency happens. Plan on how to meet or contact one another and discuss what you would do in different situations. Finally, keep this document on an easy-to-find emergency kit in case of an emergency.
2. Visit the local Council on Aging or area resources on elder abuse prevention. What are some of the resources or information you found?

References

1. Tahan, H., Watson, A., & Sminkey, P. (2016). Informing the content and composition of the CCM certification examination: A National Study from the Commission for Case Manager Certification: Part 2. *Professional Case Management, 21*(1), 3–21. https://doi.org/10.1097/NCM.0000000000000129
2. Commission for Case Manager Certification (CCMC). (2015). *Code of professional conduct for case managers*. https://ccmcertification.org/about-ccmc/code-professional-conduct
3. National Association of Social Workers (NASW). (2016). *Standards for social work practice in health care settings*. https://www.socialworkers.org/LinkClick.aspx?fileticket=fFnsRHX-4HE%3D&portalid=0
4. National Association of Social Workers (NASW). (2013). *Standards for social work case management*. https://www.socialworkers.org/LinkClick.aspx?fileticket=acrzqmEfhlo%3D&portalid=0
5. National Association of Case Managers. (2023). https://casemanagement-studyguide.com/ccm-knowledge-domains/case-management-concepts/roles-and-functions-of-case-managers-in-various-settings/
6. Institute of Medicine (US). (2001). *Committee on Quality of Health Care in America. Crossing the quality chasm: A new health system for the 21st century.* Washington DC; National Academies Press. Retrieved from: https://pubmed.ncbi.nlm.nih.gov/25057539/
7. Mottram, P., Pitkala, K., & Lees, C. (2002). Institutionalization versus-at-home long-term care for functionally dependent older people. *Cochrane Database of Systematic Reviews*, 1.
8. Carron, C. D., Ducharme, F., & Griffith, J. (2006). Deciding on institutionalization for a relative with dementia: The most difficult decision for caregivers. *Canadian Journal on Aging, 25*(2), 193–205. https://doi.org/10.1353/CJA.2006.00333
9. Legare, F., Brier, N., Stacey, D., Bourassa, H., Desroches, S., Dumont, S., Fraser, K., Freitas, A., Rivest, L. P., & Roy, L. (2015). Improving decision making on location of care with the frail elderly and their caregivers (the DOLCE study): Study protocol for a cluster randomized controlled trial. *Trials, 16*(1), 567. https://doi.org/10.1186/s13063-015-0567-7

10. United Nations. World Population Ageing. (2013). Department of Economic and Social Affairs Population Division 2013.
11. Bynum, J. P. W., Meara, E. R., Chang, C. H., Rhoad, J. M., & Bronner, K. K. (2016). *Parents, ourselves: Health care for an aging population: A report of the Dartmouth atlas project*. The Dartmouth Institute of Health Policy & Clinical Practice.
12. Weissert, W. G. (1985). Estimating the long-term care population: Prevalence rates and selected characteristics. *Health Care Financing Review, 6*(4), 83–91.
13. Ferlie, E., Challis, D., & Davies, B. (1989). *Efficiency-improving innovations in social Care of the Elderly*. Gower Publishing Ltd..
14. Department of Health and Social Services. (1990). *People first: Community Care in Northern Ireland for the 1990s*. Her Majesty's Stationery Office for DHSS.
15. Perlman, H. H. (1957). *Social casework; a problem-solving process*. University of Chicago Press.
16. McInnis, K. (2002). *Social work with elders: A biopsychosocial approach to assessment and intervention*. Allyn & Bacon.
17. Hooyman, N., & Kiyak, H. A. (2004). *Social gerontology: A multidisciplinary perspective*. Allyn & Bacon.
18. Katz, S., Down, T. D., Cash, H. R., & Grotz, R. C. (1970). Progress in the development of the index of ADL. *The Gerontologist, 10*(1), 20–30.
19. Katz, S., Ford, A. B., Moskowitz, R. W., Jackson, B. A., & Jaffe, M. W. (1963). Studies of illness in the aged-the index of ADL: A standardized measure of biological and psychosocial function. *JAMA, 185*, 914.
20. Katz, S. (1983). Assessing self-maintenance: Activities of daily living, mobility and instrumental activities of daily living. *Journal of the American Geriatrics Society (Baltimore, MD), 31*(12), 721–726.
21. Lawton, M. P., & Brody, E. M. (1969). Assessment of older people: Self-maintaining and instrumental activities of daily living. *The Gerontologist, 9*(3), 179–186.
22. American Psychological Association. (2003). *Elder abuse and neglect*. In search of solution. http://www.apa.or/pi/aging/resources/guides/elder-abuse.aspx?item=1
23. Beck, A. T., Ward, C. H., Mendelson, M., Mock, J., & Erbaugh, J. (1961). An inventory for measuring depression. *Archives of General Psychiatry, 4*, 561–571.
24. Folstein, M. F., Folstein, S., & McHugh, P. R. (1975). "Mini-mental state": A practical method for grading the cognitive state of patients for the clinician. *Journal of Psychiatry Research, 12*, 189–198.
25. Ogrin, R., Meyer, C., Karantzoulis, A., Santana, I. J., & Hampson, R. (2022). Assessing older community members using a social work tool: Developing an organizational response. *Gerontology and Geriatric Medicine.*, 8. https://doi.org/10.1177/23337214221119322
26. Whittington, C. (2007). *Assessment in social work: A guide for learning and teaching*. Author. https://www.scie.org.uk/publications/guides/guide18/
27. Berg, R. L., & Cassells, J. S. (1992). *Institute of Medicine (US) division of health promotion and disease prevention*. National Academies Press.
28. Centers for Disease Control and Prevention. (2006). https://www.cdc.gov/falls/index.html
29. Scuffham, P., Chaplin, S., & Legood, R. (2003). Incidence and costs of unintentional falls in older people in the United Kingdom. *Journal Epidemiology Community Health, 57*(9), 740–744. https://doi.org/10.1136/jech.57.9.740
30. American Geriatrics Society. (2021). https://www.americangeriatrics.org/where-we-stand/quality-patient-safety
31. Center for Disease Control and Prevention. (2015). https://www.cdc.gov/steadi/pdf/check_for_safety_brochure-a.pdf
32. Center for Disease Control and Prevention. (2012). Department of Health and Human Services. *National Institute for Occupational Safety and Health*. www.cdc.gov/noish.
33. Hasselfeld, B. W. (2023). *Benefits of Telemedicine*. Retrieved from Johns Hopkins Medicine: https://www.hopkinsmedicine.org/health/treatment-tests-and-therapies/benefits-of-telemedicine

34. Gajarawala, S. N., & Pelkowski, J. N. (2021). Telehealth benefits and barriers. *The Journal for Nurse Practitioners, 17*(2), 218–221.
35. Norman, C. D., & Skinner, H. A. (2006). eHealth literacy: Essential skills for consumer health in a networked world. *Journal of Medical Internet Research, 8*(2).
36. Arcury, T. A., Sandberg, J. C., & Bertoni, A. G. (2020). Older adult internet use and eHealth literacy. *Journal of Applied Gerontology, 39*(2), 141–150.
37. Greer, D. B., & Abel, W. M. (2022). Exploring feasibility of health to manage hypertension in rural black older adults: A convergent parallel mixed method study. *Patient Preference and Adherence*, 2135–2148.
38. Alabama Department of Human Resources. (n.d.). https://dhr.alabama.gov/adult-protective-services/
39. Peltonen, J., Leino-Kilpi, H., Heikkilä, H., Rautava, P., Tuomela, K., Siekkinen, M., et al. (2020). Instruments measuring interprofessional collaboration review. *Journal of Interprofessional Care, 34*(2), 147–161.
40. Kondrat, M. E. (2017, May 5). *Person-in-environment.* Retrieved from Oxford Bibliographies. https://www.oxfordbibliographies.com/display/document/obo-9780195389678/obo-9780195389678-0092.xml
41. Ontario Hospital Association. (2010). *Ontario Hospital Association: Quality & Patient Safety Plan (QPSP) 2010–2013*. Ontario Hospital Association.
42. Adelman, K. (2012). Promoting employee voice and upward communication in healthcare: The CEO's influence. *Journal of Healthcare Management, 57*(2), 133–148.
43. Busari, J. O., Moll, F. M., & Duits, A. (2017). Understanding the impact of interprofessional collaboration on the quality of care: A case report from a small-scale resource limited health care environment. *Journal of Multidisciplinary Healthcare*, 227–234.
44. Huang, B. Y., Cornoni-Huntley, J., Hays, J. C., Huntley, R. R., Galanos, A. N., & Blazer, D. G. (2000). Impact of depressive symptoms on hospitalization risk in community-dwelling older persons. *Journal of the American Geriatrics Society, 48*(10), 1279–1284.
45. Salanitro, A. H., Hovater, M., Hearld, K. R., et al. (2012). Symptom burden predicts hospitalization independent of comorbidity in community-dwelling older adults. *Journal of the American Geriatrics Society, 60*(9), 1632–1637.
46. Maust, D. T., Kim, H. M., Chiang, C., Langa, K. M., & Kales, H. C. (2019). Predicting risk of potentially preventable hospitalization in older adults with dementia. *Journal of the American Geriatrics Society, 67*, 2077–2084.
47. Moreno, G., Mangione, C. M., Tseng, C. H., Weir, M., Loza, R., Desai, L., Grotts, J., & Gelb, E. (2021 Jun). Connecting provider to home: A home-based social intervention program for older adults. *Journal of the American Geriatrics Society, 69*(6), 1627–1637. https://doi.org/10.1111/jgs.17071
48. Segal, E. A., Gerdes, K. E., & Steiner, S. (2013). *An introduction to the profession of social work: Becoming a change agent*. Brooks/Cole.
49. Payne, M. (2000). *Teamwork in multiprofessional care*. Bloomsbury Publishing.
50. Walrath, J. M., Dang, D., & Nyberg, D. (2010). Hospital RNs' experiences with disruptive behavior: A qualitative study. *Journal of Nursing Care Quality, 25*(2), 105–116.
51. Lapum, J., St-Amant, O., Hughes, M., & Garmaise-Yee, J. (2020). *Introduction to communication in nursing.*

Chapter 5
Skilled Nursing

Lenetra Jefferson

Learning Objectives

1. Understand how historical implications shaped the skilled nursing discipline and patient care models.
2. Classify the role of the skilled nurse in diverse care settings.
3. Discover issues that influence the nursing care of patients in diverse care settings.
4. Explain why safety considerations and crisis planning are important in the home care setting.
5. Discuss how interprofessional collaboration and team dynamics are influenced by skilled nursing contributions.

Introduction

The term *skilled nursing* has historically referred to care within a facility or nursing home setting. Yet, the ever-shifting healthcare environment, which includes the increasing use of telehealth services [1] and patients and families utilizing Internet resources for health information services [2], has not only impacted how patients and families access health but how this access influences health outcomes. Skilled nursing care is defined by HealthCare.gov [3] as services provided by licensed nurses in a home setting or nursing home setting. With the emphasis being on the *skilled* component of care, patients and their families presume competence in their

Supplementary Information The online version contains supplementary material available at https://doi.org/10.1007/978-3-031-40889-2_5.

L. Jefferson (✉)
School of Nursing, College of Health and Human Services, Troy University, Troy, AL, USA
e-mail: ljefferson150835@troy.edu

D. H. Stapleton, S. Bossie (eds.), *Home Care for Older Adults Using Interprofessional Teams*, https://doi.org/10.1007/978-3-031-40889-2_5

providers. The competency of nurses and other interprofessional team members contributes to the achievement or failure of patient care outcomes.

According to the US Department of Health and Human Services, vulnerable or underserved populations or both include older adults who are primarily serviced via skilled nursing services [4]. The basis of skilled nursing competence is understanding the framework of care and the nurse's role within it, from navigating different care environments to understanding how interprofessional collaboration and team dynamics impact patient care outcomes. Understanding and subsequently adopting a model of care for home care are central to the attainment of skilled nursing outcomes for older patients. Similarly, understanding care environments, assessment procedures, safety and crisis protocols, and interprofessional teaming is a must for those providing healthcare in the home setting.

Interprofessional Teaming and a Fundamental Care Model

It is important to remember that the patient has the center position in any given care environment. The interprofessional team and how effectively it collaborates comprise the structure supporting the patient in the center position. Honesty, helpful communication, collegiality, and appreciating the value of all team members are crucial to supporting patient care outcomes. Interprofessional collaboration requires that all team members are informed and involved in the patient care assessments, care planning, and care plan implementation. It can be argued that the greatest factor in the success or failure of home care is how well the healthcare team supports the older patient throughout the episodes of care. Research notes, "one in four Medicare patients hospitalized for acute medical illness are discharged to a skilled nursing facility (SNF); 23% of these patients are readmitted to the hospital within 30 days" [5]. Hospital readmissions are considered an assessment of failure in most healthcare systems. This outcome is also denoted as a *quality* indicator.

The interprofessional team working within the home setting must work cooperatively to meet patients' needs and to reduce hospital readmissions. This can be accomplished by communicating effectively, adhering to continuity of care standards, and including the patient and family when establishing individualized patient-centered outcomes. It can be further argued that this necessary collaboration is needed for the survival of the home healthcare environment. The nurse's role in the collaboration model of care is one of coordination and support. Physicians and advanced practice clinicians are the leaders of the care team, with the patient at the center and other members including the nurses being the framework by which the care is achieved.

The skilled nurse plays a critical role in illness management and care coordination while supporting an interprofessional approach to providing home care for patients who are older. In addition to traditional skilled nursing functions (e.g., dressing changes, wound care, blood draws and injections, intravenous (IV)

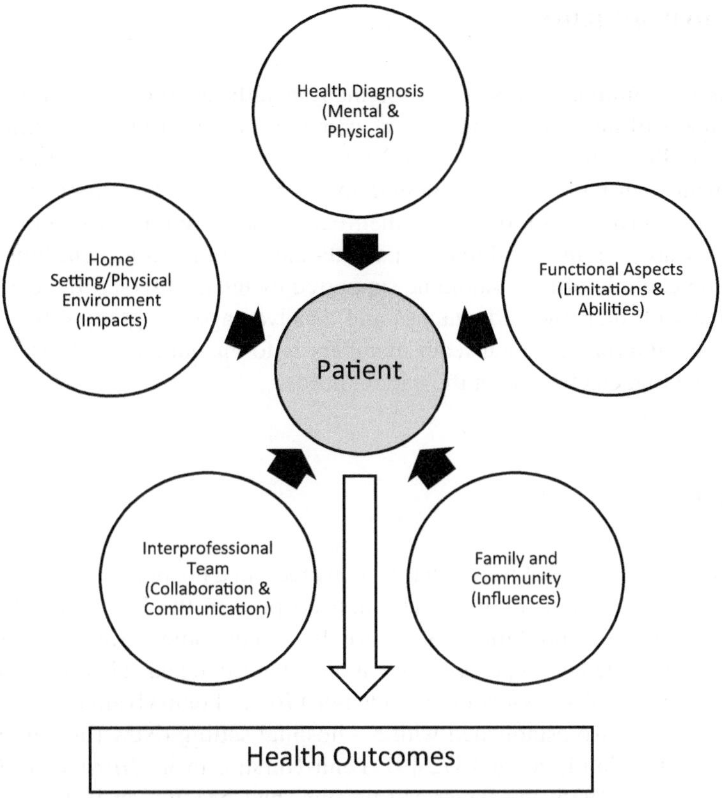

Fig. 5.1 The older patient is at the center of the care experience. This basic care model affords providers with an understanding of the many factors influencing patient health outcomes

therapy, tube feedings and other forms of nutrition, mediports), the skilled nurse frequently engages in functions that require some degree of collaboration such as care planning and participating in team conferences; assigning, delegating, and supervising; educating patients and families and interprofessional team members; acting as a patient advocate; ensuring continuity of care; and evaluating patient outcomes [6–8]. Figure 5.1 portrays a fundamental care model that has the older patient and desired outcomes as the center of the care experience. The patient's care is impacted by interprofessional teaming, health diagnoses and functional limitations, the home setting and structure, as well as specific family and community characteristics. The success or failure of patient care outcomes is dependent upon how well the skilled nurse and other team members apply this fundamental care model. The influence of these facets on patient health outcomes is well supported in the research literature.

Care Environments

Hospitals are familiar care settings for many healthcare providers. Many skilled care members of interprofessional teams commenced their training within the hospital milieu. Presently, many older patients spend less time outside of the hospital environment than within it. This population of patients is becoming increasingly focused on controlling not only how their care is delivered but where their care is delivered. Care options available to patients and families are plentiful: hospital, natural/home, clinic/office, and home supported by telehealth (see Table 5.1). They each come with their own advantages and disadvantages. A guiding best practice principle for interprofessional team members is to encourage the least restrictive environment that can best meet the patient needs.

Hospital

The traditional care model is one that is delivered via a hospital experience – traditional yes, but not from tradition. The first hospital in the USA was founded in 1751 in Pennsylvania; until then, care was delivered in home settings. The advent of facility care provided an opportunity for more supportive and scientific-based care, with the first medical school being founded in 1765 in Pennsylvania. The first nursing program was also established within a hospital setting (New England Hospital for Women and Children) in 1872 [9]. Penn Nursing in its *History of Hospitals* revealed that "by 1925, the American hospital had become an institution whose goals were recovery and cure to be achieved by efforts of professional personnel and increasing medical technology." All too often during the twentieth century, professional personnel (and not patients) were the center of care decision-making.

Clinic or Office

The clinic system is an outgrowth of the hospital environment. Today, there are clinics that function independent of hospitals and others that are structured as outpatient parts of hospital systems. Care provided in the outpatient setting is meant to be primary in nature, targeting the prevention and management of non-acute type illnesses. In recent years, clinics like hospitals have begun to adhere to the reimbursement model of care, with charting to ensure payment being a necessary focus [10].

Table 5.1 Advantages and disadvantages of care environments

Type of environment	Care environment advantages	Care environment disadvantages
Hospital setting	Access to 24/7 care Access to all members of the interprofessional team in one setting Least number of barriers for interprofessional team collaboration Potential for optimal care management, as all services are available in one central location	Potential exposure to nosocomial infections (including COVID-19) Soaring out-of-pocket costs Bells/whistles of hospital setting can lead to disorientation and confusion Care most often leads to less time for sleep and rest periods
Natural/home setting	Patients are more comfortable in their own space Care is more convenient Lower cost setting Family may be of benefit in providing care More holistic care and assessments can be conducted Increase access to healthcare Reduced travel and wait time More patient control over appointment scheduling	Persons living in home may create barriers to care Potential for lack of sleep, rest periods due to personal and/or family responsibilities or activities Potential safety risks for care providers
Natural/home setting with telehealth	Patient can feel more at ease in natural setting Home setting may aid in quality of life maintenance Increase access to healthcare Reduced travel and wait time Patients are more comfortable in their own space Care is more convenient	Access to electronic devices and the internet is limited in some communities Providers and patients must be comfortable with navigating technology Assessment may be limited due to non-face-to-face interactions
Clinic/office setting	Patient can be seen in a supported but not hospital-based care environment Cost-effective care with a primary care focus Possible access to members of the interprofessional team in one setting	Potential exposure to nosocomial infections Increase in focus on number of patients seen to maximize reimbursement; limits provider with patient time Typically, Monday–Friday office hours

Natural or Home

The origin of medical care is deeply rooted in the natural or home setting. Before formal medical training programs, care was often delivered by natural healers or members of Christian societies. Skilled nursing also has its genesis in the natural or home setting. The idea of a "health visitor" originated with Florence Nightingale [11], but others, such as Harriet Tubman, are often overlooked when discussing the history of the nursing profession and a natural-based care framework. The University of Virginia's Maura Singleton in *Flashback Friday – Harriet Tubman's Overlooked Story as a Nurse* [11] revealed how Ms. Tubman provided care to soldiers in addition to rescue efforts on behalf of enslaved Americans. Tubman traveled to South Carolina in 1862 to provide nursing care and education to the Gullah in their natural/home environment. The Gullah were enslaved descendants from West and Central Africa.

Telehealth

Telehealth is becoming the option of choice for a selection of patients and providers. Although telehealth has been around for a while, access and demand for this care option are increasing. Previously known as telemedicine, hospitals would use it as a way to deliver health via a closed-circuit system within the facility. In April 2020, during the first surge of COVID-19 cases, it accounted for 69% of doctor-patient visits [12]. This rise in telehealth's use was necessitated by the pandemic, but it now embodies a practical framework for effective care practices.

Skilled in the Home Care Setting

Skilled nurses are ever present in the home environment, providing the necessary skills, expertise, and support. They are available 24/7 via nurse chat lines offered through clinics or hospitals or via visits supported by home health networks. Nursing support can be the difference between successful illness management and failure. An assessment of the physiological aspects of patients (as well as environmental, social, and psychological factors) is needed to ensure effective home care delivery. A care approach based on a health assessment framework is underscored in foundational courses required of nursing students. The home itself and the infrastructure within all warrant a skilled nursing assessment.

Nursing Assessment in the Home Care Environment

The patient assessment is the initial phase of skilled nursing care. The assessment comprises a data collection process and utilizes a holistic approach including physiological, psychological, socioeconomic, and cultural components [13]. The assessment of an older patient comprises additional considerations [14] as listed in Table 5.2. Notable areas of assessment pertain to activities of daily living, functional status, cognitive functioning, and mobility. The results are useful in determining a patient's ability to care for self and environment (self-sufficiency), a patient's quality of life, and a patient's degree of cognitive decline.

Furthermore, the patient assessment must identify current needs and potential future needs. There are several tools that can be utilized within the home setting to delineate patient needs. The Outcome and Assessment Information Set (OASIS) [15] is a popular home environment assessment tool. This standard assessment tool was designed to ensure that assessment data is appropriately linked to patient care outcomes. Additional versions (e.g., OASIS – C, D, and E) have been published since the original 1999 release. Nurses and other team members must guarantee that data is collected in a systematic manner to promote accurate assessment of patients' care needs. If the skilled nurse encounters any atypical assessment data, the supervising physician or advanced practice personnel, advanced practice registered nurse (APRN), or physician assistant (PA) should be contacted. Well-coordinated home visits by skilled nurses are fundamental when assessing aging-related risks and spearheading collaborative efforts to address and reduce these risks [16, 17]. Regularly scheduled skilled nursing home visits may positively influence the provision of successful home assessments and ultimately patient outcomes.

Table 5.2 Assessing the older patient in the home care environment

Focus	Description
Activities of daily living	The skilled nurse (in conjunction with other IP team members) assesses ability to complete daily activities including bathing, dressing, toileting, grooming, and feeding
Functional status	The skilled nurse (in conjunction with other IP team members) assesses ability to manage finances, transportation needs, shopping, and grocery needs
Cognitive functioning	The skilled nurse (in conjunction with other IP team members) assesses cognitive ability by using established cognitive clinical assessments
Mobility	The skilled nurse assesses mobility functions within and external to the home structure, particularly movements to necessary appointments and social endeavors

Safety Considerations and Crisis Planning

Skilled nurses and members of the interprofessional team must implement safety measures in the home setting to guarantee practice standards are met and patient outcomes are attained. The success or failure of care is dependent on multiple factors as discussed in Fig. 5.1. Yet, safety for both the patient and home care provider is always paramount and can have a bearing on patient outcomes. Before venturing out from the hospital and clinic environment (which is relatively protected), the nurse must become adept at assessing the home milieu for health and safety concerns. Home care providers have limited control over the home setting (e.g., cleanliness, maintenance of infection control standards, pets, who has access to the home, etc.). Similarly, the provider has no control over neighborhood or community dynamics. In a survey conducted by the National Nurses United (2021), nearly half (48%) of hospital nurses reported a small or significant increase in workplace violence [18]. The potential for workplace violence in the home setting should always be assessed. The workplace extends to any environment in which the skilled nurse is providing care. Table 5.3 describes health and safety risk factors that may pertain to the patient and the healthcare provider [19]. The nurse, as one of the designated leaders of the interprofessional team, should always explore these risk factors with the patient and family to determine their impact on health and recovery. The family should be assisted in developing reasonable solutions or options. The nurse should transparently disclose to the interprofessional team any health and safety risk factors that are identified within the home setting.

Safety planning in the home environment should encompass planning for potential crises. In acute care settings, interprofessional team members are expected to take on assigned roles during times of crisis. The same type of anticipatory planning must occur in the home setting, and team members should be very transparent about safety concerns presented or observed in the home setting. The interprofessional team should convene routinely to discuss potential crises from man-made disasters, to weather-related disasters, to pandemic-focused events. Designated team members should enact safety and crisis plans as needed. Planning and executing routine crisis exercises can best create a proactive way to manage the potential effects of crises [20].

Chapter Summary

This chapter has discussed the role of the skilled nurse as an interprofessional team member. Additionally, the author underscored the importance of operating within a care framework that accentuates the recognition and adoption of a fundamental care model. Understanding how the environment affects health outcomes is a crucial aspect in navigating the home healthcare experience. This chapter discussed the advantages and disadvantages of the various care environments. Assessment as the

Table 5.3 Health and safety risk factors [19]

Risk factor	Examples
Threats of violence and abuse	Elder abuse or maltreatment
	Neighborhood violence
	Overt prejudice and discrimination
	Drug use
	Gun use
Environmental threats	Threatening neighbors
	Threatening family members
	Threatening clients
	Threatening pets
Slips/trips/falls	Clutter in the home
	Loose rugs/slippery floors
	Loose or uneven floorboards
	Poor lighting
Environmental hazards	Animal hair
	Excessive dust
	Peeling paint
	Mold and dampness
	Poor air quality
	Temperature extremes
	Loud noises
	Obstructing furniture
Potential chemical/medical hazards	Irritating chemicals
	Poisons
	Hazardous smells
	Misuse or overuse of medications
Unsanitary conditions	Insects, bugs
	Rodents
	Unhygienic conditions

initial point of care delivery along with recommendations for safety and crisis planning was also discussed. Additionally, the reader was provided a few best practice guidelines for interprofessional collaboration. It is important to remember that each member plays a necessary and valuable role in supporting patients and families and in maximizing health outcomes.

A Skilled Nurse's Response to the Case Study on Jeralean

When reviewing the circumstances of Jeralean, the skilled nurse must first remember that Jeralean, as the patient, is always the center of care. We also have to remember that we do not work in silos and that the team approach works best to support the attainment of optimal care outcomes. With Jeralean as the center of our care approach, the first step would be for the nurse (per physician's directive) to contact all members of the team. Once this contact is established, a meeting should be called to begin the process of working with Jeralean and her daughter, Alice. During this initial meeting, Jeralean and Alice should be encouraged to provide an update on health status, concerns, and needs. This update should occur prior to developing the patient's plan of care. Care goals and objectives must be established with the patient's active participation and with team members delineating their roles and the purpose of proposed interventions. Jeralean and Alice should be encouraged and supported in asking questions and must give consent to the interventions. Consideration should be given to scheduling services at times that are convenient and respectful of the family events. Team members should provide their contact information (email and phone numbers) and communicate (to all) the best time to receive calls or emails. Team members should commit to communicating timely and transparently with Jeralean, with Alice, and with each other. The team must remain in regular contact to ensure that Jeralean's care goals are met and that her quality of life is enhanced. This first meeting should be the first of many dialogs, whether in-person, via phone, or via a virtual meeting. Because the nurse often has the most contact with the family and the prescribing physician, this member of the interprofessional team should actively commit to keeping everyone "in the know," resolving communication roadblocks, and ensuring the continuity of care.

Discussion Question

1. What is the role of the skilled nurse on the interprofessional team?

Multiple Choice Questions

1. What are the priorities that should be established when assessing a patient's home during the initial visit?
   (a) Determine the pharmacy of choice
   (b) Ask the physician what they want should be done
   (c) Assess physical environment, and establish patient care needs and expectations
   (d) Determine how best to conduct the home visit
2. You are visiting your patient in the home setting for the third visit, and the patient tells you "my legs just keep getting weaker, the older I get." Which of the following would be the best action to take?
   (a) Consult with your team leader for a physical therapy assessment

(b) Ask the patient to walk throughout the house for an assessment
(c) Tell the patient, “no worries, this is expected as you get older”
(d) Continue with your assessment and care

3. Which of the following clinicians are not considered interprofessional team members? Select all that apply.

(a) The provider (MD, APRN, PA)
(b) The nurse
(c) The social worker
(d) The home health aide
(e) The patient

4. When describing skilled nursing care, which of the following is not considered to be an essential component?

(a) Services from licensed nurses at the hospital
(b) Services from licensed nurses at home or in a nursing home
(c) Care services from therapists or technicians in the home
(d) Care services from aides or other assistive personnel in the home or facility

5. Which of the following is an advantage of the home care (natural) setting?

(a) Persons living in home may create barriers to care
(b) Potential for lack of sleep or rest periods due to personal and/or family responsibilities or activities
(c) Potential safety risks for care providers
(d) Patient can feel more at ease in natural setting

References

1. U.S. Government Accountability Office. (2022, September 29). *Telehealth in the pandemic – How has it changed health care delivery in medicaid and medicare?* https://www.gao.gov/blog/telehealth-pandemic-how-has-it-changed-health-care-delivery-medicaid-and-medicare
2. Patel, V., & Johnson, C. (2019). *Trends in individuals' access, viewing and use of online medical records and other technology for health needs: 2017–2018.* The Office of the National Coordinator for Health Information Technology.
3. Healthcare.gov. (n.d.). *Skilled nursing care.* https://www.healthcare.gov/glossary/
4. U.S. Department of Health and Human Services. (n.d.). *Serving vulnerable and underserved populations course.* https://www.hhs.gov/guidance/sites/default/files/hhs-guidance-documents/006_Serving_Vulnerable_and_Underserved_Populations.pdf
5. Britton, M., Ouellet, G., Minges, K., Gawel, M., Godshon, B., & Chaudhry, S. (2017). Care transitions between hospitals and skilled nursing facilities: Perspectives of sending and receiving providers. *The Joint Commission Journal on Quality and Patient Safety, 43*, 565–572.
6. Interprofessional Professionalism Collaborative. (2018, August 15). *IPC case scenario for Mr. Jones part I.* [Video]. YouTube. All rights reserved. https://youtu.be/woHaclEtLFw
7. Interprofessional Professionalism Collaborative. (2019). *IPA tool kit.* http://www.interprofessionalprofessionalism.org/toolkit.html

8. NURSA. (2023). *Skilled nursing specialty: The ultimate guide to SNF jobs*. https://nursa.com/specialties/skilled-nursing
9. University of Pennsylvania School of Nursing. (2011). *History of Hospitals*. https://www.nursing.upenn.edu/nhhc/nurses-institutions-caring/history-of-hospitals/
10. American Hospital Association. *Current and emerging payment models*. Retrieved from https://www.aha.org/advocacy/current-and-emerging-payment-models
11. Singleton, M. (2019). *Flashback Friday- Harriet Tubman's Overlooked Story as a Nurse*. https://www.nursing.virginia.edu/news/flashback-harriet-tubman-nurse/
12. Pearl, R., & Wayling, B. (2022). The Telehealth Era is just beginning. *Harvard Business Review*. https://hbr.org/2022/05/the-telehealth-era-is-just-beginning
13. American Nursing Association. (n.d.). *The nursing process*. https://www.nursingworld.org/practice-policy/workforce/what-is-nursing/the-nursing-process/
14. University of Michigan. (n.d.). *Geriatric functional assessment*. https://www.med.umich.edu/lrc/coursepages/m1/HGD/GeriatricFunctionalAssess.pdf/pogoe.org/sites/default/files/geriatric_functional_assessment_module.pdfhttps:/hign.org/consultgeri-resources/elearning
15. Ohio Department of Health. (n.d.). *Outcome and Assessment Information Set (OASIS)*. https://odh.ohio.gov/know-our-programs/outcome-and-assessment-information-set-oasis/outcomeandassessmentinformationsetoasis#:~:text=The%20Outcome%20and%20Assessment%20Information,maternity%20home%20health%20care%20patients
16. Tay, Y., Abu Bakar, N., Tumiran, R., Ab Rahman, N., Areefa, N., Ma'amor, A., Yau, W., & Abdullah, Z. (2021). Effects of home visits on quality of life among older adults: A systematic review protocol. *Systematic Reviews, 10*, 1–7. https://doi.org/10.1186/s13643-021-01862-8
17. Fulmar, T., Reuben, D., Auerbach, J., Fick, D., Galambos, C., & Johnson, K. (2021). Actualizing better health and health care for older adults. *Health Affairs, 40*(2). https://doi.org/10.1377/hlthaff.2020.01470
18. National Nurses United. (2022). *National nurse survey reveals significant increases in unsafe staffing, workplace violence, and moral distress*. https://www.nationalnursesunited.org/press/survey-reveals-increases-in-unsafe-staffing-workplace-violence-moral-distress
19. Gershon, P., Pogorzelska, M., Quresahi, K., Stone, P., Canton, A., Samar, S., Westra, L., Damsky, M., & Serman, M. (n.d.). Home health care patient & safety hazards in the home: Preliminary findings. *Agency for healthcare Research & Quality, 1*.
20. Institute for Healthcare Improvement. (n.d.). *Crisis management*. https://www.ihi.org/resources/Pages/ViewAll.aspx?FilterField2=IHI_x0020_Topic&FilterValue2=d1f5d356-9e8d-4610-87e0 e007323999bb&Filter2ChainingOperator=And&TargetWebPath=/resources&orb=Created

Chapter 6
Physical Therapy

Gilaine Nettles, Revenda Greene, Ashley Cancer, and Bridgette Stasher-Booker

Learning Objectives

1. Comprehend the role and responsibilities of the physical therapist and physical therapist assistant in the home healthcare setting.
2. Acquire knowledge to facilitate the evaluation of the client's needs in the home environment.
3. Accentuate traditional assessment procedures in the home environment.
4. Identify safety considerations and related crisis planning necessary when treating clients in the home care environment.
5. Explain the interprofessional collaboration and referrals necessary to ensure appropriate coordination of medical services.
6. Recognize the role of the healthcare provider in the provision of telehealth/telemedicine services.
7. Understand the interprofessional team dynamics and the role of the physical therapist in the case study of Jeralean.

Supplementary Information The online version contains supplementary material available at https://doi.org/10.1007/978-3-031-40889-2_6.

G. Nettles (✉) · R. Greene · A. Cancer
Department of Physical Therapy, College of Health Sciences, Alabama State University, Montgomery, AL, USA
e-mail: gnettles@alasu.edu; revenda.greene@gmail.com; acancer@alasu.edu

B. Stasher-Booker
Department of Health Information Management, College of Health Sciences, Alabama State University, Montgomery, AL, USA
e-mail: bbooker@alasu.edu

D. H. Stapleton, S. Bossie (eds.), *Home Care for Older Adults Using Interprofessional Teams*, https://doi.org/10.1007/978-3-031-40889-2_6

Introduction

Physical therapy is a critical component of interprofessional care. This medical treatment facilitates successful recovery and rehabilitation after surgery, illness, or injury. Physical therapists (PTs) are highly trained healthcare providers who specialize in movement analysis and dysfunctions and help patients regain the functional independence necessary to maintain quality of life. PTs are considered *movement experts*. Physical therapy interventions can help to reduce the impact, severity, and duration of an illness or injury and help prevent the long-term consequences of disabilities and chronic diseases [1].

Home health physical therapy allows patients to return to their prior levels of daily activities, i.e., work, leisure and recreational activities, doctors' appointments, and community activities. PTs and their trained and licensed physical therapist assistants (PTAs) work to help patients who are older restore their mobility, understand their health conditions, and meet their physical needs safely within the natural home environment. To obtain licensure to practice, PTs and PTAs must graduate from an accredited institution of higher education, pass a national licensure examination, and maintain this license in the state jurisdiction in which they practice. PTs instruct patients and caregivers on methods to accomplish the desired results through therapeutic interventions such as exercise regimens, modalities for pain management, home adaptations, and gait training with or without supported equipment.

Interprofessional rehabilitation teams typically include physicians, rehabilitation nurses, physical therapists, occupational therapists, speech and language pathologists, clinical psychologists, social workers, dieticians, prosthetists, and rehabilitation engineers [2]. The PT's role on the interprofessional team is to identify, diagnose, and treat movement problems and to restore and maximize movement. PTs also help patients to manage symptoms such as pain using exercise and other modalities. PTs strive to help patients who are older regain their highest level of physical function, participate in their normal daily activities, and maintain as much physical independence as possible. PTs develop specific goals and design interventions for each patient based on the patient's goals for physical functions and movement. PTs and PTAs work with older patients and their caregivers to empower them to make personal decisions about the outcome of their home care experiences. Older patients are encouraged to take an active role in each therapy session, from the beginning to the end [3].

The PT uses a framework called the *patient client management model* for patient care, which entails the following: [3].

- Examining the patient
- Evaluating findings of examination data
- Developing a physical therapy diagnosis of the impact of the patient's condition on their physical function and movement

- Formulating a prognosis which is a prediction of the anticipated outcome and the amount of time required to reach the optimal level of function
- Designing and implementing a plan of care to reach the desired goals and expected outcomes
- Determining the interventions or methods of treatment, techniques, and procedures to achieve the desired results; and
- Reexamining the patient to determine the effectiveness of the interventions in achieving the expected outcomes

Natural Environment Versus Office Setting (Juxtaposition of Risks and Benefits)

Many patients prefer to age in place and desire the ability to function independently in their homes and natural environments as long as possible. According to the 2021 Home and Community Preference Survey by the American Association of Retired Persons, 80% of adults aged 50 and older want to remain in their homes and communities as they age [4]. Sixty percent of older adults own their own homes; and approximately one-third of them report that they need to modify their homes as they get older for mobility and safety reasons.

A 2020 study on the impact of physical therapy on Medicare beneficiaries with a primary diagnosis of dementia reported that patients' functional skills improved with home health visits, with the rate of progress being proportional to the number of visits by the PT. The researchers reported a 25.3% greater probability of improving activities of daily living (ADLs) functions with physical therapy services. The researchers also reported that these patients have greater difficulty accessing outpatient therapy (office/clinic) services and are less likely to adhere to the outpatient appointment schedule [5]. The World Health Organization (WHO) defines adherence as "the extent to which a person's behavior corresponds with agreed upon recommendations from a health care provider" [6]. Transportation and environmental factors that reduce safety with ambulation and mobility and adversely impact adherence with scheduled outpatient appointments are not factors in the home care setting. A 2009 article entitled "Barriers to Treatment Adherence in Physiotherapy Outpatient Clinics: A Systematic Review" found that factors such as depression, anxiety, poor support systems, and low physical activity levels result in low outpatient treatment adherence [7]. These aspects can be more effectively addressed in the home healthcare milieu.

Accentuating Traditional Assessment Procedures and Evaluating Needs

When PTs begin home health interventions, they assess the home for barriers that could hinder functional activities or present safety hazards. The therapist begins the service with recommendations that reduce safety hazards and prevent falls and other accidents. Safety assessments are used to help therapists determine if environmental barriers exist and recommend modifications to reduce the barriers. Examples of safety assessment instruments include the Home and Community Environment (HACE) assessment of mobility and the Environmental Analysis of Mobility in the home [8]. These assessments provide a quantitative score as a baseline for the home assessment that enables the therapist to reassess safety and mobility after modifications are made in the home [9].

Moreover, PTs use home assessment checklists and performance-oriented assessments of mobility to determine a patient's safety, balance, gait, and mobility [8]. Preventing falls is one of the primary goals of PT home assessments. Performance-based measurements are used to examine functional mobility skills. These measurements also produce a quantitative score that can be compared with industry norms for patients by age and by diagnoses. Examples of these performance-based measures include the Timed Up and Go Test (TUG), the Tinetti or Performance Oriented Mobility Test, and the Berg Balance Assessment [7].

Initial Interview

A detailed interview is the initial step to commencing physical therapy services with the older patient in the home care environment. This detailed interview of the patient and the caregiver is a central component of the PT evaluation. During the interview, the PT attempts to understand the patient's prior level of functioning in various settings and activities; the social, family, and medical history; past injuries, hospitalizations, and surgeries; and current and past medications and treatment interventions [10, 11]. The initial interview and patient observations include an assessment of the following:

- History of falls
- Environmental safety and awareness
- Cognitive status
- Use of assistive devices and adaptive equipment in the home and community
- Communication skills and hearing impairments
- Visual impairments
- Incontinence with bowel or bladder function
- Medication interactions, compliance, number of different medications and prescribers
- Medications that may increase fall risks [11]

The PT works closely with the patient, the caregiver, and other interprofessional team members to obtain information that will allow the practitioner to choose the best treatment interventions, equipment, and course of action to optimize function and safety in the home care setting. Medicare, a federal health insurance for people 65 or older, requires a physician certification of a patient's homebound status as a prerequisite to receiving therapy services at home [10]. Medicare regulations mandate written evidence of the need for assistance from a third party, the need for mobility aids like wheelchairs or walkers, and the need for special transportation to appointments outside of the home. Medicare regulations also stipulate that in order to receive physical therapy services, there must be a documented need for such services to maximize a patient's functional outcomes. According to Medicare, only licensed PTs or PTAs can perform *skilled* physical therapy services [12].

Outcome and Assessment Information Set (OASIS)

Medicare regulations require a complete home assessment, the Outcome and Assessment Information Set (OASIS). The OASIS is a mandatory assessment for Home Health Agencies (HHA) and a condition for participation in the Medicare Home Health Program sponsored by the Centers for Medicare and Medicaid Services (CMS), a federal agency under the Department of Health and Human Services. The OASIS includes sociodemographic information and a comprehensive examination of the patient's prior functional status and the current level of function in all activities of daily living (bathing, grooming, dressing, toileting, transferring, ambulation and locomotion, feeding and eating, planning and preparing meals, transportation, laundry, housekeeping, shopping, and telephone usage) [13]. Since 1999, the OASIS data sets have evolved to include more specific outcome measures. The most current version of the OASIS is the OASIS-E. RNs and PTs are responsible for completing the OASIS documentation to initiate the care plan for each episode of care for home health patients. See Appendix C for a view of an interactive interprofessional assessment form (adaptable to OASIS) that can be used by interprofessional team members [20].

Patient Examination

After completing a thorough interview, the PT examines the patient. A physical therapy examination incorporates reviewing the systems and particular tests and measurements to gather factual baseline information about the patient. The PT examines the skin, heart, lungs, muscles, bones, joints, and nervous system. A thorough review of these systems enables the therapist to make decisions about the treatment plan and expected outcomes for the patient. The information gleaned from the examination serves as a basis for ruling out potential health conditions, consulting with other interprofessional team members, and referring to providers and programs more appropriate to the care needs of the patient. The PT evaluates the patient and tracks development over time using a variety of valid and reliable tests and measurements. Tests and measures are necessary to confirm a physical therapy diagnosis by ruling in or out the specific causes of physical limitations and impairments [11]. These tests and measurements include, but are not limited to, the following:

- Joint range of motion measurements using a goniometer
- Manual muscle strength tests and functional mobility skills
- Endurance tests with activities such as walking, with and without assistive devices
- Skin and wound assessments
- Cardiovascular and pulmonary function tests to determine stamina, blood pressure, pulse, respiratory rate, and oxygen saturation rates with physical activities
- Screening of other body systems, such as gastrointestinal, renal, mental, and cognitive functions, to rule out potential complications and make referrals as needed [11]

The examination concludes with the gathering of information about the patient and the evaluation of baseline information. The PT then lists significant concerns related to physical function, disability, and health. Once the diagnosis is confirmed, the therapist develops a prognosis that includes a plan of care designed to improve function by providing interventions to address the list of needs. The plan of care is designed to help return the patient or client to their optimal functional status [3, 11]. The WHO created the International Classification of Functioning, Disability, and Health (ICF) framework to ensure that healthcare professionals use the same terminology when discussing illnesses and functional impairments [14].

PTs are trained to evaluate the data from the systems review and tests and measures and synthesize them in the International Classification of Function context. The ICF framework enables the therapist to prioritize the impairments, activity limitations, and participation restrictions; address the environmental and personal factors to determine the relationships; and make clinical decisions relating to diagnosis, prognosis, interventions, and expected outcomes. PTs develop a care plan with the patient and caregiver and communicate routinely with the interprofessional team. Each member of the healthcare team completes a similar assessment process. Providing elder care conjointly with an interprofessional team in the natural environment can reduce healthcare costs for the patient and society [11]. The patient management of care model adopted by most PTs comprises examination, evaluation, diagnosis, prognosis, intervention, and outcome components. The primary components of care include examination, evaluation, diagnosis, prognosis, intervention, and outcomes.

Referrals/Selecting Care Personnel/Coordinating Medical Services

The PT presents to the interprofessional team a physical therapy/rehabilitation diagnosis that conveys the impact of the health condition on the client's physical function. PTs and other healthcare providers use the ICF framework to communicate the findings of their professional examinations based on their training, roles, and responsibilities to other team members. Interprofessional team members review the clinical evaluations of all providers before developing a plan of care and establishing a prognosis for the patient. The frequency and duration of physical therapy services is determined in conjunction with the patient, the caregiver, and interprofessional team members [11].

In many cases, the PT and the registered nurse (RN) lead the development of the interprofessional team's care plan. This occurs subsequent to the physician and nurse providing a medical diagnosis based on an evaluation of the pathology, lab values, and other tests to determine the disease or disorder at a cellular level. The PT should collaborate regularly with the patient's occupational therapist, speech therapist, social worker, nursing assistant, and other medical specialists, if applicable.

Gougeon et al. (2017) discussed how teams can offer significant expertise in the natural environment to permit older patients to remain at home. Their study reviewed four randomized controlled trials and four nonrandomized controlled clinical trials in Canada to assess the effectiveness of interprofessional (IP) healthcare models. The study revealed that IP teams have a significant positive impact on patient quality of life and care satisfaction. The researchers determined that more research on interprofessional team dynamics is needed to better appreciate the impact of team training, collaborative behavior, team culture, and treatment implementation processes on home healthcare for older patients. An increased awareness of these dynamics will contribute to the implementation of best practices that will render important measurable outcomes relating to reductions in hospitalizations, emergency room visits, and home health visits [2].

Safety Considerations and Crisis Planning

Physical therapists in the home environment may be employed by a home care agency or may be self-employed independent contractors working directly for patients. Because they have little control over their work environment, they may be exposed to several safety and health hazards. These hazards include blood-borne pathogens and biological hazards, latex sensitivity, ergonomic hazards from patient lifting, violence, hostile animals, and unhygienic and dangerous conditions [15]. In addition, if their daily work schedule requires them to provide care for multiple patients, they face hazards on the road as they drive from home to home.

Physical therapists often assist patients with mobility skills such as transfers to various surfaces, including from the bed to a wheelchair, ambulation with assistive devices, and learning how to use the bathroom with walkers, crutches, or canes. The act of moving and lifting patients can result in injuries for healthcare providers and patients.

A hazard review was published by the National Institute for Occupational Safety and Health (NIOSH) to educate the public on risks associated with home health care and preventive measures to decrease injuries and even deaths in home healthcare. NIOSH has also produced factsheets on home health risks. Some of the factsheet topics are listed below [15].

- Sprains and strains
- Exposure to unsafe work conditions
- Preventing workplace, on-the-job violence
- Driving-related incidents
- Needlestick prevention
- Latex allergies
- Musculoskeletal injuries
- Self-care while caring for others

Telehealth in Home Healthcare

Since the start of the COVID-19 pandemic, telerehabilitation has increased as a substitute for face-to-face home health services. Telehealth in rehabilitation, also known as telerehabilitation, refers to the provision of consultation services, preventive care, and diagnostic and therapeutic services via technology from a remote location. Health-related quality of life and functional outcomes achieved by veterans who received home health PT services via telehealth and in-home video have been examined [16]. Researchers used a pre- and post-design study to assess 26 veterans who received services via the Rural Veterans Telerehabilitation Initiative (RVTRI). They concluded that those enrolled in the telerehabilitation initiative avoided nearly 3000 miles in travel to the outpatient clinic and $1151 to $1326 in travel reimbursement by utilizing the real-time, home-based, physical therapy telerehabilitation service [16]. These services have increased veterans' access to healthcare, particularly in rural areas, reduced health disparities, and reduced the cost of treatments and the number of emergency room visits [16].

Telehealth has been embraced throughout the profession of physical therapy, and the American Physical Therapy Association has issued the following position statement:

> Telehealth is a well-defined and established method of health services delivery. Physical therapists provide services using telehealth as part of their scope of practice, incorporating elements of patient and client management as needed, to enhance patient and client interactions. The American Physical Therapy Association (APTA) supports:

- inclusion of physical therapist services in telehealth policy and regulation on the national and state levels to help society address the growing cost of health services, the disparity in the accessibility of health services, and the potential impact of health workforce shortages;
- advancement of physical therapy telehealth practice, education, and research to enhance the quality and accessibility of physical therapist services; and,
- expansion of broadband access to provide all members of society the opportunity to receive services delivered via electronic means.
(APTA, *Advocacy Issues/Telehealth*, 2021) [17]

The Role of the Physical Therapist Assistant

The physical therapist assistant (PTA) works under the supervision of a licensed PT to help patients recover from injuries or illnesses that affect their ability to move and function. The role of a PTA includes implementing treatment plans, monitoring patient progress, assisting with therapeutic procedures, educating patients and caregivers, and maintaining equipment. The PTA assists in the implementation of treatments designed by the PT, including exercises, stretches, and other therapeutic interventions to help patients regain their strength, mobility, and flexibility. While implementation of the plan of care is the primary focus, PTAs also observe and document the progress of the patient's recovery and report back to the PT about any changes or concerns [18]. PTAs assist with various therapeutic procedures, such as heat or ice therapy, electrical stimulation, and massage. They teach patients how to perform exercises and activities correctly to maximize their recovery. The PTA is responsible for maintaining and cleaning equipment used in physical therapy sessions [19]. Overall, a PTA plays a vital role in helping patients recover from injuries or illnesses by providing hands-on support and working collaboratively with PTs to develop and implement treatment plans that meet the unique needs of each patient [19].

Chapter Summary

This chapter explained the role of the physical therapist and physical therapist assistant in providing home care services on an interprofessional team. Physical therapy is a crucial component of the rehabilitation process, and PT interventions are required to help patients regain functional independence necessary to maintain quality of life. This chapter explored the provision of physical therapy in the natural environment, the use of telehealth services in the home setting, and the home assessment procedures and documentation required for Medicare. This chapter also discussed the safety concerns in the home and ways physical therapy can help minimize safety hazards and increase functional independence with home modifications and the use of adaptive equipment. Readers were introduced to the relationships between the interprofessional team members and how the physical therapist collaborates with the team to help achieve patient-centered goals and objectives. Lastly, the authors demonstrated the responsibilities of the PT and discussed team dynamics, referencing the case study introduced in Chap. 3.

The Interprofessional Team Dynamics Case Study: Jeralean

Because Jeralean is concerned with having "too many doctors" and being on "too many medications," she would benefit from a case manager to manage her health status. Case managers are healthcare professionals who serve as patient advocates to support, guide, and coordinate care for patients, families, and caregivers as they navigate their health and wellness journeys. Because Jeralean's daughter is unable to coordinate her care effectively, the case manager's expertise would be of benefit. Jeralean may also benefit from virtual visits to health professionals, so she would be less overwhelmed with input from health professionals.

Skilled physical therapy services are indicated for this client. The PT should address the client's functional strength and mobility and develop a plan of care to address strength and mobility deficits, especially because the patient has experienced a recent and significant decline in her functional status. The PT should also request or reach out to the following professionals to address health concerns and to increase the probability of Jeralean being able to age at home with dignity:

Nursing tech or home health aide (under the supervision of a skilled registered nurse): A home health aide is needed because of the client's decreased strength, visual deficits, and difficulty managing medication. The home health aide would assist with ADLs and IADLs (bathing, feeding), arrange medication and ensure that the patient takes her medication daily, measure insulin correctly and administer shots as indicated, and perform light housekeeping so that the patient can maintain a clean household and avoid injuries.

Occupational therapist (OT): The OT is needed to facilitate independence in ADLs and IADL (grooming and self-care, feeding, bathing) and to evaluate the client's cognitive status to determine if she can reside in her home safely or benefit from placement in an assisted living facility.

Registered dietician nutritionist (RDN): The RDN is needed to evaluate the patient's diet and provide patient education for Jeralean and her daughter to ensure that the patient's diet is sufficient to facilitate the healing of wounds.

Social worker (SW): The SW is needed to address the patient's depression and identify possible community services she may be eligible for, such as Meals on Wheels. However, these services may not be available because the client resides in a rural region.

There is an urgent need for the establishment of a home health team. The client is at significant risk for a further decline in her health, medical, and functional status if a home health team is not established and activated to prevent the decline.

Discussion Question

1. Considering the APTA Guide to Physical Therapy Practice, during which step(s) should interprofessional communication take place, and what information must be shared relevant to the step(s) identified?

Multiple Choice Questions

1. Which of the following statements is *true* about physical therapists?
   (a) Physical therapists are considered movement experts
   (b) PTs help patients to regain the functional independence necessary to maintain their quality of life.
   (c) PT interventions can help to reduce the impact, severity, and duration of an illness or injury
   (d) All of these statements are true.
2. Physical therapists treat patients with physical therapist assistants. Which of the following statements is *false* about PTAs?
   (a) PTAs are licensed by the State Board of Physical Therapy in the jurisdiction in which they practice.
   (b) PTAs must graduate from an accredited institution of higher education with a PTA program
   (c) Physical therapist assistants must be supervised by a licensed physical therapist.
   (d) Physical therapist assistants are trained on the job by physicians, PTs, or nurses.
3. Physical therapists use a framework for patient care called the *patient client management model*. The *patient client management model* includes which of the following components?
   (a) Examination, evaluation, diagnosis, prognosis and plan of care, interventions, and outcomes
   (b) Plan of care, home assessments, performance-based measures and interventions for safety
   (c) Therapeutic exercises, fall prevention, patient education
   (d) Interventions, outcomes, diagnosis, and prognosis
4. Which of the following statements is *true* regarding older patients?
   (a) Older patients are more likely to live with their children after 65 years of age.
   (b) The majority of older patients aged 50 and older want to remain in their homes and communities as they age.
   (c) Older patients have difficulty adhering to home health appointments.
   (d) Older patients tend to prefer to go to outpatient clinics for physical therapy.

5. In order to reduce fall risks, the physical therapist works with the patient and caregiver and the interprofessional team to ensure that the home environment is safe. Which of the following is considered a safety hazard in home healthcare?
   (a) Lifting and moving patients
   (b) Clutter and throw rugs on the floors
   (c) Pets and hostile animals on the property
   (d) All of these are considered safety hazards

References

1. Sahrmann, S. (2022). Doctors of the movement system – Identity by choice or therapists providing treatment – Identity by default. *International Journal of Sports Physical Therapy, 17*(1). https://doi.org/10.26603/001c.30175
2. Gougeon, L., Johnson, J., & Morse, H. (2017). Interprofessional collaboration in health care teams for the maintenance of community-dwelling seniors' health and well-being in Canada: A systematic review of trials. *Journal of Interprofessional Education & Practice, 7*, 29–37. https://doi.org/10.1016/j.xjep.2017.02.004
3. American Physical Therapy Association. (2022). *Guide to physical therapist practice 4.0*. APTA Store. https://store.apta.org/guide-to-physical-therapist-practice-3-0.html
4. Binette, J. (2021a, 2021). Home and community preferences survey: A national survey of adults age 18+ – methodology. *AARP*. https://doi.org/10.26419/res.00479.004
5. LeDoux, C. V., Lindrooth, R. C., Seidler, K. J., Falvey, J. R., & Stevens-Lapsley, J. E. (2020). The impact of home health physical therapy on medicare beneficiaries with a primary diagnosis of dementia: A secondary analysis of Medicare data. *Journal of the American Geriatrics Society, 68*(4), 867. https://doi.org/10.1111/jgs.16307
6. WHO. (2003). *Adherence to long-term therapies: Evidence for action*. World Health Organization. https://archive.org/details/adherence_full_report
7. Jack, K., McLean, S. M., Moffett, J. K., & Gardiner, E. (2010). Barriers to treatment adherence in physiotherapy OUTPATIENT CLINICS: A systematic review. *Manual Therapy, 15*(3), 220–228. https://doi.org/10.1016/j.math.2009.12.004
8. Gitlin, L. N. (2003). Conducting research on home environments: Lessons learned and new directions. *The Gerontologist, 43*(5), 628–637. https://doi.org/10.1093/geront/43.5.628
9. O'Sullivan, S., Schmitz, T., & Fulk, G. (2019). Chapter 9 examination of the environment. In *Physical rehabilitation* (6th ed., pp. 338–393). F A DAVIS.
10. Medicare.gov. *What's medicare?* https://www.medicare.gov/what-medicare-covers/your-medicare-coverage-choices/whats-medicare. Accessed 22 Jan 2023.
11. O'Sullivan, S. B., et al. (2019). Chapter 1 clinical decision-making and examination. In *Physical rehabilitation* (7th ed., pp. 1–18). McGraw-Hill Education LLC.
12. CMS. (2021, April). *Medicare home health benefit booklet – hhs.gov*. Health and Human Services. https://www.hhs.gov/guidance/sites/default/files/hhs-guidance-documents/MLN908143_2020_05_Medicare_Home_Health_Benefit_Booklet_Final.pdf.
13. Center for Medicare and Medicaid Services. (2022) *Outcome Assessment Information Set Version E (OASIS-E)*. https://www.cms.gov/files/document/oasis-e-guidance-manual51622.pdf.
14. World Health Organization. 2001. *The International Classification of Functioning, Disability, and Health (ICF)*. Geneva: WHO. http://www.who.int/classifications/icf/en/
15. U.S. Department of Labor. (2022). *Department of Labor United States Department of Labor*. Home Healthcare – Overview | Occupational Safety and Health Administration. https://www.osha.gov/home-healthcare.

16. Levy, C. E., Silverman, E., Jia, H., Geiss, M., & Omura, D. (2015). Effects of physical therapy delivery via home video telerehabilitation on functional and health-related quality of life outcomes. *Journal of Rehabilitation Research and Development, 52*(3), 361–370. https://doi.org/10.1682/jrrd.2014.10.0239
17. APTA. (2021, November 17). Position Paper: Expanded Telehealth Access Act of 2021. *APTA, Advocacy Issues.* www.apta.org/advocacy/issues/telehealth/expanded-telehealth-access-act-of-2021.
18. Clynch, H. M. (2023). *The role of the physical therapist assistant: Regulations and responsibilities* (2nd. ed.). F.A. Davis Company.
19. American Physical Therapy Association. (2022). *Guide to physical therapist practice 4.0.* APTA Store. https://store.apta.org/guide-to-physical-therapist-practice-3-0.html.
20. Kim, S. Y. (2017). Continuity of care. *Korean Journal of Family Medicine, 38*(5), 241. https://doi.org/10.4082/kjfm.2017.38.5.241

Chapter 7
Occupational Therapy

Lovett Lowery, Letitia Osburn, Jessica Maxwell, Dailen Castillo, and Kenya Crews

Learning Objectives

1. Identify and discuss the occupational therapist's role in providing home care services.
2. Explore the provision of occupational therapy services in the natural environment, and juxtapose it to the provision of occupational therapy services in the clinic or office setting.
3. Identify and discuss ways to use the home environment to accentuate and strengthen traditional assessment procedures.
4. Discuss issues faced by older individuals related to safety considerations and emergency preparedness in the home.

Supplementary Information The online version contains supplementary material available at https://doi.org/10.1007/978-3-031-40889-2_7.

L. Lowery (✉)
Alabama State University, Montgomery, AL, USA
e-mail: llowery@alaasu.edu

L. Osburn · K. Crews
Department of Physical Therapy, College of Health Sciences, Alabama State University, Montgomery, AL, USA
e-mail: kcrews@alasu.edu; losburn@alasu.edu

J. Maxwell
School of Physical Therapy, University of the Incarnate Word, San Antonio, TX, USA
e-mail: jmaxwell@uiwtx.edu

D. Castillo
College of Physical Therapy, University of Incarnate Word, San Antonio, TX, USA
e-mail: dccastil@uiwtx.edu

D. H. Stapleton, S. Bossie (eds.), *Home Care for Older Adults Using Interprofessional Teams*, https://doi.org/10.1007/978-3-031-40889-2_7

5. Understand how interprofessional collaboration is practiced in home care services as an alternative for continued medical care of older adults.
6. Discuss how occupational therapy services are integrated into an interprofessional collaborative team to serve older adults needing home healthcare services.
7. Identify how occupational therapy referrals are generated in an interprofessional collaborative team.
8. Explore occupational therapy's role in care coordination of medical services and care personnel.
9. Discuss how telehealth services are beneficial in home care services and how they are used in the incorporation of occupational therapy services.

Occupational Therapy

Occupational therapy (OT) is one of several health professions among the interprofessional team that provide home care services for the older population. It is "the therapeutic use of everyday life occupations with persons, groups, or populations for the intent of improving or supporting participation and engagement in one's daily occupation" [1]. In occupational therapy, occupations refer to "the everyday activities that people do as individuals, in families, and with communities to occupy time and bring meaning and purpose to life. Occupations include things people need to, want to and are expected to do" [2]. "Occupational therapy practitioners use their knowledge of the transactional relationship among the client, the client's engagement in valuable occupations, and the context to design occupation-based intervention plans" [1]. With the emergence of home care service provision and the increasing older population, it is important to ensure that this particular client population can live and age in the home setting safely and productively. With the use of occupations and the therapeutic use of self as the cornerstones of the profession and emphasis on the client's occupations, contexts, performance patterns, performance skills, and other client factors as OT's domain of practice, occupational therapy practitioners are equipped to serve this growing population and facilitate older adults' engagement in meaningful and purposeful activities. Its "practitioners provide community-based services to people throughout the lifespan," and "community can serve as both the setting of occupational therapy for an individual as in the home, but also as the focus of the intervention" [1]. In this chapter, we will explore the OT's role in providing home care services, as well as the provision of occupational therapy services in the natural environment. We will also juxtapose the provision of occupational therapy services in the natural environment to that in a clinic or office setting. This chapter will explore ways to use the home environment to accentuate and strengthen traditional assessment procedures. Safety concerns, crisis planning, and the use of telehealth services by OTs will also be discussed.

Natural Environment Versus Office Setting (Juxtaposition of Risks and Benefits)

The quality of OT services provided is just as important as the location where they are being provided. Environmental factors include the physical, social, and attitudinal surroundings of where people live and/or conduct their lives while also influencing the function and disability of individuals [3]. Environmental factors that can influence the function and disability of individuals include positive aspects to facilitate and negative aspects that serve as barriers or hindrances [4]. Many benefits come from both natural environments and the office settings while focusing on engaging clients in activities of daily living (ADLs), instrumental activities of daily living (IADLs), health management, rest/sleep, education, social participation, work, play, and leisure [1]. The aim of both settings is to select, create, modify, and use the physical environment to facilitate health, well-being, and participation in the desired occupations of patients and clients [5]. This section will focus on the risks and benefits of each occupational therapy service environment.

There are federal policies and legislation that support occupational therapy's role in shaping social contexts and environments to facilitate and promote participation in occupations and health and wellness [5]. Natural environment and human-made changes to the environment animate and inanimate the components of the natural or physical environment for the betterment of the clients [3]. Natural environments can include settings such as the person's home, work, school, community spaces, grocery store, and other places. Natural environments are settings that are natural or normal for individuals without disabilities.

Natural environments are real-life environments unlike simulated environments that are made to resemble and replicate natural environments in the office or clinical setting. Natural environments consist of settings where routines and daily activities are carried out. These places are where everyday tasks are performed and where natural social interactions and events occur. Participating in naturally occurring activities in their rightful environment serves as good learning opportunities that promote knowledge acquisition and development. Working with families in the natural environment is also important when training to become an OT. Individuals learn best by watching families interact with each other and how they do things, thus promoting family participation [5]. Natural environments better accommodate typical client routines and activities. These environments provide opportunities to identify supports and barriers to care that are not discernable in office settings. Lastly, within clients' natural settings, the OT can create individual treatment plans based upon daily habits and routines, natural tools, and readily available resources. The OT can recommend adjustments and home modifications to promote safety and functioning and decrease risk of falls. A risk of providing care in a natural environment is that the OT is usually alone when implementing evaluations and treatments; thus, the treatment intervention will be based on what the OT can assist the client with independently.

Simulated office environments are a unique approach to treatment that can provide immersive yet safe space to support therapy with the potential to assist a wide range of individuals [6]. Simulated environments in office settings are artificially created environments that give patients and clients a simulated experience that can be used to diagnose and treat psychological conditions that cause difficulties for patients. These environments are the next best thing to natural environments when patients are in clinical care and unable to receive therapy at home. Although simulated environments can aid in offering patients the opportunity to practice activities that could transfer to their natural environments, natural environments still provide the best opportunity for treatment. Natural environments render natural artifacts, noises, smells, and spaces that simulated environments cannot provide. Simulated environments can risk patients' injury at home (e.g., attempting to perform a task in a support office environment; yet the natural environment may be limited in resources, rearranged differently than the office, and may even have animals that cause tripping hazards). Simulated environments can offer patients false hope of being able to accomplish the same tasks the same way in their home environments. Simulated office environments tend to be more structured and safer than natural environments that are not set up by OTs. The benefit of providing OT services in the office setting is having on-hand support from other therapists for lower-level patients who fatigue easily and would benefit from co-treating with other therapy services due to the level of dependency, among other things.

Accentuating Traditional Assessment Procedures and Evaluating Needs

Home environments are perfect contexts for assessments and treatments. Accentuating traditional assessment procedures and evaluating the needs of clients within their homes offer the opportunity to gather rich and comprehensive information. The OT evaluation process focuses on understanding what the client wants and needs to do; determining what the client can do or used to do; and identifying the necessary supports and what barriers or limitations are present to promote health, wellness, and participation [3]. Home environments offer unique and intimate opportunities to work in a natural environment without having to recreate the client's context.

Evaluating clients within their homes can offer many benefits for the patient and opportunities for the therapist. Implementing traditional assessment procedures and evaluations within the client's home can aid in improving efficiency and optimizing patient outcomes. Within the home environment, safety measures and other treatment plans can center around the natural environment, equipment/tools, and sounds among other things to successfully increase the carryover of the goals. The home environment is the most natural environment to implement traditional assessment procedures. Assessing daily habits and routines is also easier to assess and address within the home environment. Within the home environment, OT assessments can range from taking vital signs, rearranging furniture for safety, implementing equipment, and assessing ADLs such as bathing, dressing, feeding, grooming, and toileting and IADLs such as cooking, cleaning, washing dishes, sweeping, laundry, and medication management [1]. OTs can also observe and assess clients' level of functioning and safety while performing transfers to the toilet, chairs, bed, and shower chair while also performing ADLs.

Safety Considerations and Crisis Planning

According to the Centers for Disease Control and Prevention (CDC), more than 30 million older adults sustain falls yearly, resulting in more than 30,000 deaths [7]. More than 2.5 million older adults are treated annually in emergency departments for fall injuries [7]. Falls markedly are noted as significant factors in impacting the ability of older clients. Falls can result in decreased daily activity participation and overall quality of life [8]. Most falls occur in older adults' homes [9]. For this reason, older adults need to become cognizant of environmental hazards to include those unique to home design. Safety considerations and crisis planning for home safety in older adults may be beneficial in decreasing the statistical inferences mentioned above.

Implementing color contrast in an older person's environment can assist with home orientation while facilitating navigation [10]. As individuals age, their visual acuity decreases, and perceptual changes occur, which creates visual ambiguity in their depth perception, visual memory, and figure-ground perception [10]. Enhancing an older adult's environment by increasing lighting, reducing glare, maximizing contrast, and removing hazards can improve visual functioning [11].

Many homes have probable dangers directly related to the following: unsteady furniture, impeded footpaths, insufficient lighting, and unsecured rugs. The previously listed hazards are integral facets connected to increased fall risks for older adults living at home [12]. Adaptive environments and durable medical equipment can promote functional independence while serving as safety measures for older adults living at home. Because high cost may be associated with environmental home adaptations, this mediating factor requires the OT to recommend minimal and no-cost solutions. Before incorporating environmental changes, it is essential to ascertain acceptance from the older adult. It is equally vital to thoroughly explain the benefits of incorporating environmental modifications with attention to the financial demands placed on the client [9].

In the wake of natural disasters across the nation, it is essential for older adults living at home to have emergency preparedness awareness. Older individuals' emergency preparedness can diminish due to physical and cognitive challenges; therefore, support-service providers, including OTs or caregivers, are pivotal in establishing an emergency plan for this population. This emergency plan should contain contact listing information for emergency personnel, family members, and close associates. According to the CDC, older adults should have a list of prescriptions, allergies, a 3-day minimal medication supply, vendor information for all medical devices, medical documents, hearing devices, additional batteries, and visual aids, including glasses and contacts, as a primary disaster supply kit [13].

The overall theme of safety considerations and crisis planning for older adults in the home environment as it relates to occupational therapy is for practitioners to facilitate a functional environment by addressing environmental factors and enhancing occupational performance. By targeting occupations and intervention strategies that increase independence in self-care management, identification of potentially hazardous situations, and developing, managing, and maintaining health and wellness routines, OTs are helping to establish healthy performance patterns and skills that will enhance the safety of older adults living at home.

Interprofessional Collaboration

Due to the COVID-19 pandemic, home healthcare has been more common and an encouraged alternative for continued medical care of older adults. Older adults requiring home care services usually suffer from multiple comorbidities putting them at risk of requiring various healthcare services and interventions. To facilitate a safe and successful transition home for the patient, a collaborative approach must be supported between different healthcare professionals and healthcare providers. Therefore, promoting an interprofessional team provides a climate where it is essential to understand the collaboration within and across the healthcare services to prevent fragmentation of care and promote holistic healthcare. Interprofessional collaboration in home care involves focusing on the patients' needs, taking the collaborative relationship into account, and having a reflective and questioning approach to improve the patients' quality of life. Having this attitude fosters a feeling of "trust and security" and a "flexible and critical approach without boundaries between multiple caregivers" [14].

The key to success in home care is "flexibility and improvisation" [14]. An interprofessional treatment approach is viable in order to meet the needs of older adults living at home to address complex situations and medical conditions. An interprofessional team approach cultivates a collaborative environment where multiple caregivers can deliver their skills and competencies to treat older adults requiring home care services due to multiple comorbidities. Common and achievable goals set by the interprofessional team pertain to assessing, planning, performing, and evaluating patient care. Furthermore, working with a collaborative team helps promote open communication and encourages a shared decision-making methodology in home care [14]. Additionally, it is suggested that "effective interdisciplinary teamwork has a more positive influence on patient outcome than other quality improvement strategies" [14].

Integration of Occupational Therapy into an Interprofessional Collaborative Team

OT services are among several possible services provided for older adults needing healthcare services while living at home. The integration of occupational therapy services into an interprofessional collaborative team is well supported by the American Occupational Therapy Association (AOTA). AOTA affirms that occupational therapy practitioners are trained to be direct care providers, consultants, educators, case managers, and advocates for clients and their families [15]. In addition, the American Occupational Therapy's Association's Vision 2025 supports occupational therapy services interprofessional partnership between occupational therapy and "all people" to be necessary to "maximize health, well-being, and quality of life" [16]. OT practitioners have a unique insight into the significant impact that occupations have on "health and wellness" making their contribution to patient care valuable [17]. OT practitioners receive comprehensive training to deliver evidence-based practice that addresses the whole person, making them qualified to work effectively within interprofessional collaborative teams. Their holistic perspective allows them to be effective both as interprofessional healthcare team members and as direct care providers to support client, family, and community needs in traditional and emerging settings [1]. As a result, AOTA recognizes that OT practitioners are well prepared to contribute to interprofessional collaborative care teams in multiple settings to address the needs of individuals across all life spans [1].

OT practitioners provide several services to include evaluation and intervention strategies to the older adult while addressing contextual aspects of health, medication management, psychosocial implications, cognition, lifestyle modification, environmental barriers, and safety [15]. Working within the interprofessional model, an OT's role is to interact, collaborate, and coordinate with the team and develop an individual plan of care tailored to the patients' needs. OT practitioners work collaboratively with interprofessional teams supporting each healthcare provider to provide the highest level of care for the older adult [15].

OT Referrals in an Interprofessional Collaborative Team

OT practitioners have extensive training addressing the person-environment-occupation in multiple settings to facilitate optimal function, engagement, participation, and health [18]. Due to the diversity in areas of practice that occupational therapy can address, therapists can be consulted to service older adults in home care struggling with complex health needs and provide patient-centered care. According to AOTA [17], occupational therapy also has a distinct role in addressing mental health and behavioral health as they pertain to occupational performance. Occupational therapy practitioners have the capacity to recommend additional healthcare services by initiating a referral to the attending physician and recommend treatment of musculoskeletal conditions or mental health conditions. Furthermore, OT practitioners are also able to make recommendations pertaining to adaptive equipment/devices, environmental/behavioral modification, and safety awareness within a home setting environment [1, 16].

Care Coordination of Medical Services and Selecting Care Personnel

As one of the healthcare service providers in home care, an OT coordinates services with other service providers and families. The occupational therapy education "focuses on patient and caregiver education; psychosocial, physical, cognitive, cultural, and environmental, therefore occupational therapy practitioners are equipped for collaboration with other medical services" [19, p. 503]. OT practitioners have extensive training working in a variety of areas that encompass patient and caregiver education, psychosocial, physical, cognitive, cultural, and environmental areas. They demonstrate the critical skills, education, and competencies necessary to coordinate medical services in home care in an interprofessional collaborative team. The central theme supporting occupational therapy in care coordination is the concept of patient and family needs, preferences, and the expertise of the team members [19]. The occupational therapy practitioner has the ability to collaborate with team members and match services to patient and family needs by completing screening and evaluation, assessment, coordination of care, and transitional care.

Telehealth

According to the Centers for Disease Control and Prevention "telehealth is the use of communications technologies to provide health care from a distance" [20]. Telemedicine has also been used for decades in clinical settings [21]. We all acknowledge that COVID-19 turned the world we once knew upside down. There was global panic and healthcare systems were overwhelmed. It was during the bleakest points of the pandemic that telehealth came to the rescue. Will we now witness healthcare systems transitioning to wide-ranging use of telehealth? Of course, there are limitations, barriers, advantages, and benefits to the use of this healthcare option. Many of these have been discussed in previous chapters. Research has posited that telehealth services can prevent disparities and rectify access issues in healthcare. It has been stated that "when some people have access to that new knowledge and expertise and other people do not, disparities grow" [21]. It has been further postulated that "advanced telecommunication and information technologies have a role to play in transforming the healthcare system" [21]. Evidence-based models facilitated by these technologies can improve healthcare access and quality across the geographic and economic spectrum [21]. This is great news for stakeholders. Patients, their families, and interprofessional team members will all benefit from telehealth services. It has been concluded that telehealth was underused and understudied until the COVID-19 pandemic [22]. Thus, throughout COVID-19, occupational therapists (early adopters of telehealth) were able to hone their skills through the innovative use of the telehealth medium. Telehealth is an impactful public health intervention with the potential to significantly improve care access for underserved populations, become an acceptable and quality standard of care, improve provider-patient bonds, and reduce healthcare costs [23].

Case Study: Occupational Therapy Practice Framework

The Occupational Therapy Practice Framework (OTPF), which consists of the OT domain and process, "describes the central concepts that ground occupational therapy practice and builds a common understanding of the basic tenets and vision of the profession" [1]. The "profession's understanding of the domain and process of occupational therapy guides practitioners as they seek to support clients' participation in daily living, which results from the dynamic intersection of clients, their desired engagements, and their contexts" [1]. Many healthcare professions use a similar process of evaluating, intervening, and targeting outcomes [1]. The OT domain can be used to enhance the understanding of occupational therapy's unique role in interprofessional team collaboration and its contribution to team dynamics.

Occupational Therapy Domain

The aspect of the OTPF that we will focus on in this section is the occupational therapy domain. It assists in identifying the client's occupations, contexts, performance patterns, performance skills, and client factors. It also helps in connecting different components related to the client and how it affects the client's performance in day-to-day tasks. Therefore, it is essential for occupational therapy practitioners to know and understand the OT domain, as well as its importance. "This knowledge sets occupational therapy apart as a distinct and valuable service" [1]. The following sections will explore how the OT domain is incorporated in our client case study, through our look at Jeralean's occupations, contexts, performance patterns, performance skills, and other client factors (see Table 7.1).

Table 7.1 Applying aspects of the occupational therapy domain to the case study

	Occupations	Contexts	Performance patterns	Performance skills	Client factors
Case study application: Jeralean	**ADLs:** showering, grooming, hygiene	**Environmental:** home environment	**Habits:** gets out of bed daily, sits on couch, noncompliant with medication	**Motor:** grips, manipulates, moves, transports	**Values/ beliefs:** none specified, low motivation/ volition
		No assistive or adaptive equipment		**Process:** chooses, uses, handles, initiates, organizes	
	IADLs: housekeeping, cooking				**Body functions:** multiple body functions affected
			Routines: walking	**Social interaction:** approaches, looks, discloses, expresses emotions	**Body structures:** multiple body structures affected
	Health management: medication management, nutrition management	Travels for healthcare services	**Roles:** mother, previously wife, co-caregiver		
		Daughter resides with her			
		Personal: 75-year-old			
		African American			
	Rest and sleep: sleep routine	Recent widow			
	Social participation: Previously quite social				

Occupations

Jeralean is an older woman who presents with multiple medical complexities and physical impairments that affect her engagement in her everyday occupations. There are nine occupations within the OT domain, and some of Jeralean's occupations include activities of daily living (ADLs), instrumental activities of daily living (IADLs), health management, rest and sleep, and social participation. More specifically, she is noted to be very meticulous about grooming and self-care and maintained a neat and orderly home. Although she is not compliant with wearing her prosthesis, this is an important area of dressing. All of these are related to the occupations ADLs and IADLs. Because of her multiple medical conditions, Jeralean states she takes too much medication and is noncompliant with her medication regimen. This area of care is addressed under the occupation health management, and OT can assist in medication management, as well as health management occupations such as physical activity, nutrition management, and personal care device management. One occupation not often considered is rest and sleep, which involves sleep preparation and sleep participation. Jeralean is exhibiting difficulty with falling asleep and remaining asleep at night and may benefit in establishing an environment conducive to rest and sleep and developing routines to prepare for sleep. Because she was once quite social, Jeralean is limited in another occupation, social participation, due to a limited social outlet. Occupational therapy can assist her in engaging in activities that involve social interactions with others. All of these occupations mentioned can be used in the occupational therapy process as a targeted outcome for the client, but also as a therapeutic tool to achieve the targeted goals.

Contexts

In relation to Jeralean's contexts, her environmental factors include all the aspects of her "physical, social, and attitudinal surroundings" [1] in which she lives that affect her function. Therefore, the OT practitioner must take into consideration Jeralean's home environment, her relationship with her daughter, Alice, and the support she provides. Jeralean's context can be either an enabling or inhibiting factor to her engagement in her occupations. Jeralean lives in her natural environment, at home with her daughter. However, despite her many health conditions, Jeralean home is not near any health facilities, and she must travel over 60 miles to receive healthcare services. She is noted to have had several falls in different areas of her home and does not have any adaptive equipment or wheelchair. So, her physical environment and availability of resources and equipment may be an inhibiting factor. But in contrast, the support of her daughter, who is in good health and who prioritizes caregiving of her mother, is a factor that will help to enable Jeralean's participation in her day-to-day occupations. Another aspect of her context the OT practitioner must consider is Jeralean's personal factors. "Personal factors are internal influences affecting functioning and disability" that "reflect the essence of the person" [1]. These factors provide more insight into who Jeralean is beyond the state of her health and may include her chronological age, life experiences, social background, character traits, education, and lifestyle. The OT practitioner may note that Jeralean is a 75-year-old African American woman who was active in activities in her home and socially engaged until the recent loss of her husband less than 1 year ago. Since her husband's passing, Jeralean has shown a decrease in her occupational engagement, as well as changes in her interests and level of motivation.

Performance Patterns

The past and present performance patterns of Jeralean are also identified by the OT. These include any acquired habits, routines, roles, or rituals Jeralean used when participating in her daily occupations. "OT practitioners" who consider clients' past and present behavioral and performance patterns are better able to understand the frequency and manner in which performance skills and health and unhealthy occupations are, or have been, integrated into clients' lives. Some habits and shared routines Jeralean previously engaged in were daily walks with her husband, shared household tasks, and cooking. However, after her husband's death, it is notable that Jeralean consumes an unhealthy diet and exhibits a change in her sleeping habits. The passing of her husband has also changed her role as a wife, and despite being a parent, the roles in the relationship with her daughter are affected with her declining health.

Performance Skills

"Performance skills are observable, goal-directed actions that result in a client's quality of performing desired occupations" [1]. There are three types of performance skills that the OT can address, and they include motor skills, process skills, and social interaction skills. There are numerous skills contained within this section, but not all are addressed in an OT treatment session or throughout the duration of care. These performance skills contribute to the occupational performance for a client. For example, Jeralean is noted to have an issue with dropping glasses and plates because they slip out of her hand. Although there are different performance skills that can be addressed, one performance motor skill that may be identified by the OT practitioner as an area of concern is grips or manipulates. Jeralean exhibits balance issues that may be related to other performance motor skills, as well as difficulty with her medication that may be related to performance motor or process skills. Her decreased social engagement may be related to deficits in social interaction skills. Despite the performance skills affected, effective use of performance skills contributes to how an occupation is carried. Adaptations or assistive equipment may be required to assist or compensate for the loss of a performance skill.

Client Factors

"Client factors include values, beliefs, and spirituality; body functions, and body structures that reside within the client and influence the client's performance in occupations" [1]. This is an important aspect to consider. An individual's values and spirituality contribute to how the client views oneself and his or her situation.

Although Jeralean's values and beliefs are not specifically mentioned in the case study, it is important to note that she exhibits low motivation and volition. Exploring this aspect of the OT domain could prove beneficial in motivating Jeralean in her health journey and be an enabling support to achieve her occupational outcomes.

Chapter Summary

Understanding occupational therapy's domain of practice gives greater insight into OT's role in the interprofessional team's dynamics in the provision of home care services. Rendering services in the home care setting affords the profession of occupational therapy to hone in on the client's occupational performance in his or her natural environment. When working with an interprofessional team, occupational therapy's unique use of occupations as a means to an end as well as a therapeutic tool provides the opportunity to address the client holistically and make a collaborative effort to facilitate positive client outcomes.

The profession of occupational therapy is founded on the therapeutic use of occupations to achieve purposeful and meaningful patient outcomes. The OT's contribution of evaluating the client's need and implementing occupation-based interventions is supported in the individual-client environment. In the home care setting, great consideration can be given to the client's as well as their caregiver's interests, safety considerations, and crisis preparation. What better location to provide occupational therapy services and address real-life goals, barriers to progress, patient resources, etc. than in the client's natural (home) environment? With occupational therapy's emphasis on the therapeutic use of occupation and the use of the natural environment to accentuate intervention, home care services for the population of older adults offer innumerable, real-life opportunities in the provision of quality occupational therapy services, along with other disciplines of the interprofessional team, to facilitate client engagement in everyday occupations. In accordance with AOTA's Vision 2025 statement, the profession of occupational therapy is dedicated to partnering with other healthcare professions to ensure a collaborative effort in assisting the client to live life at his or her maximum potential, including in the home environment.

Discussion Questions

1. What is the occupational therapist's role in the provision of home care services?
2. How does the occupational therapist use the home environment in accentuating the assessment of a client's needs?
3. Discuss how the profession of occupational therapy supports the integration of interprofessional partnerships.

Multiple Choice Questions

1. Natural environments are more disruptive for clients than the office location because they are built into the client's daily routines and are supportive for the client and his or her families as they participate in everyday activities.
   (a) True
   (b) False
2. Which of the following supports occupational therapy services interprofessional partnership between occupational therapy and "all people" to be necessary to "maximize health, well-being, and quality of life"? Choose the best answer.
   (a) AOTA's Code of Ethics
   (b) AOTA's Vision 2025
   (c) AOTA's Mission
   (d) None of the above
3. The following public health tool is often defined as the use of communications technologies to provide healthcare from a distance.
   (a) Teleporting
   (b) Telephone communications
   (c) Telehealth
   (d) Telegram
4. Older adults need to consider the environmental factors of their homes, including environmental obstacles and design factors. All, except which of the following, are safety considerations that may assist older adults in their home environment? Please choose the best answer.
   (a) Adding color contrast
   (b) Increasing lighting
   (c) Removing clutter
   (d) Adding decorative rugs
5. Which of the following healthcare professions emphasize the therapeutic use of everyday life occupations for the intent of improving or supporting participation and engagement in one's daily occupation?
   (a) Speech therapy
   (b) Occupational therapy
   (c) Physical therapy
   (d) Behavioral therapy

References

1. American Occupational Therapy Association. (2020a). Occupational therapy practice framework: Domain and process (4th ed.). *American Journal of Occupational Therapy, 74*(2). https://doi.org/10.5014/ajot.2020.74S2001
2. World Federation of Occupational Therapists. (2012). *About occupational therapy*. Retrieved from https://www.wfot.org/about-occupational-therapy
3. American Occupational Therapy Association. (2020b). Policies supporting OTs role in shaping contexts and environments. *American Journal of Occupational Therapy.* https://www.aota.org/advocacy/everyday-advocacy/ots-role-in-shaping-contexts-and-environments
4. Giraldo-Rodriguez, L., Mino-Leon, D., Murillo-Gonzalez, J. C., & Agudelo-Botero, M. (2019). Factors associated with environmental barriers of people with disabilities in Mexico. *Revista de saude publica, 53*, 27. https://doi.org/10.11606/S1518-8787.2019053000556
5. American Occupational Therapy Association. (2021). Occupational therapy scope of practice. *American Journal of Occupational Therapy, 75*(Suppl. 3), 7513410020. https://doi.org/10.5014/ajot.2021.75S3005
6. Muller, R. T. (2019). *Simulated environments provide new treatments for mental problems.* https://trauma.blog.yorku.ca/2019/11/simulated-environments-provide-new-treatments-for-mental-health-problems/
7. Centers for Disease Control Prevention. (n.d.). *Keep on your feet-preventing older adult falls.* https://www.cdc.gov/injury/features/older-adult-falls/index.html
8. Mortazavi, H., Tabatabaeichehr, M., Taherpour, M., & Masoumi, M. (2018). Relationship between home safety and prevalence of falls and fear of falling among elderly people: A cross-sectional study. *Journal of the Academy of Medical Sciences of Bosnia and Hertzegovina, 30*(2), 103–107. https://doi.org/10.5455/msm.2018.30
9. Bonder, B., & Wagner, M. (2001). *Functional performance in older adults* (2nd ed.). F.A. Davis Company.
10. Cooper, B. (1985). A model for implementing color contrast in the environment of the elderly. *The American Journal of Occupational Therapy, 39*(4).
11. Dirette, D., & Gutman, S. (2021). *Occupational therapy for physical dysfunction* (8th ed.). Wolters Kluwer.
12. Lord, S., Menz, H., & Sherrington, C. (2006). Home environment risk factors for falls in older people and the efficacy of home modifications. *Age and Ageing, 35*(2), 55–59. https://doi.org/10.1093/ageing/afl088
13. Centers for Disease Control Prevention. (n.d.). *Emergency preparedness for older adults.* https://cdc.gov/aging/publications/features/older-adult-emergency.html
14. Larsen, A., Broberger, E., & Petersson, P. (2017). Complex caring needs without simple solutions: The experience of interprofessional collaboration among staff caring for older persons with multimorbidity at home care settings. *Scandinavian Journal of Caring Sciences, 31*(2), 342–350.
15. American Occupational Therapy Association. (2020c). Role of occupational therapy in primary care. *American Journal of Occupational Therapy, 74*(Suppl.3), 7413410040p1.
16. American Occupational Therapy Association. (2016). *AOTA unveils Vision 2025.* Retrieved from https://wwwaota.org/aboutaota/vision-2025.aspx
17. American Occupational Therapy Association. (2020d). Occupational therapy in the promotion of health and Well-being. *American Journal of Occupational Therapy, 74*, 7413410010. https://doi.org/10.5014/ajot.2020.743003
18. Ainsworth, L., & de Jonge, D. (2014). The relevance and application of universal design in occupational therapy practice. *Occupational Therapy Now, 16*(5), 5–7.
19. Moyers, P. A., & Metzler, C. A. (2014). Health policy perspectives-interprofessional collaborative practice in care coordination. *American Journal of Occupational Therapy, 68*, 500–505. https://doi.org/10.5014/ajot.2014.685002

20. Centers for Disease Control and Prevention. (2020). *The use of telehealth and telemedicine in public health*. Updated July 8, 2020. https://www.cdc.gov/publications/topic/telehealth.html. Accessed 20 Sep 2020.
21. Nesbitt, T. S. (2012, August). The evolution of telehealth: where have we been and where are we going. In *The role of telehealth in an evolving health care environment: Workshop summary*. Institute of Medicine.
22. Shaver, J. (2022). The state of telehealth before and after the COVID-19 pandemic. *Primary Care: Clinics in Office Practice, 49*(4), 517–530.
23. Marcoux, R. M., & Vogenberg, F. R. (2016). Telehealth: Applications from a legal and regulatory perspective. *Pharmacy and Therapeutics, 41*(9), 567–570.

Chapter 8
Behavioral Healthcare

Danita H. Stapleton and Sekeria Bossie

Learning Objectives

1. Understand aspects influencing behavioral health in late life.
2. Recognize causes of mental illness or psychological distress in individuals who are older.
3. Discuss various interventions designed to improve the behavioral health of older adults.
4. Implement interventions designed to improve the behavioral health of older adults.

Introduction

The older adult population continues to grow. Over the past 10 years, the number of adults over the age of 65 increased by 33% [1]. These numbers are projected to almost double by 2060 [1]. Population projections indicate that by 2030, all baby boomers (people born in the years 1946–1965) will be older than age 65 [2, 3]. According to the US 2017 Census Report [1]:

> Between 2016-2040, the number of individuals 85 years old and over are projected to increase by 129%. Persons reaching age 65 are expected to live on average an additional 19.4 years (20.6 years for females and 18 years for males). Older women (27.5 million)

Supplementary Information The online version contains supplementary material available at https://doi.org/10.1007/978-3-031-40889-2_8.

D. H. Stapleton (✉) · S. Bossie
Department of Rehabilitation Studies, College of Health Sciences, Alabama State University, Montgomery, AL, USA
e-mail: dstapleton@alasu.edu; sbossie@alasu.edu

D. H. Stapleton, S. Bossie (eds.), *Home Care for Older Adults Using Interprofessional Teams*, https://doi.org/10.1007/978-3-031-40889-2_8

> outnumber older men (21.8 million). About 28% (13.8 million) of persons over the age of 65 live alone. Of those aged 75 and over, nearly half of women, (45%) live alone. Between 2016 and 2030, the white (not Hispanic) population age 65 and over is projected to increase by 39% compared to 89% for older racial and ethnic minority populations, including Hispanics (112%), African Americans (not Hispanic) (73%), American Indian and Native Alaskans (not Hispanic) (72%), and Asians (not Hispanic) (81%).

Not only is it essential for interprofessional team members to comprehend the significance of the aforementioned statistics; it is similarly important that they understand that this population often exhibits emotional, mental, and behavioral health concerns. One study revealed that 35% of older individuals had been diagnosed with a mental disorder ($N = 400$) [4]. The researchers also found a significant correlation between mental health and gender, education, coexistence type, job, and chronic diseases ($p < 0.001$). As a result of their findings, they underscored the importance of initiating meaningful educational programs to bring awareness to relative and predictive factors that can improve health and reduce the prevalence and development of mental disorders in older adults. The most common conditions include anxiety, severe cognitive impairment, and mood disorders such as depression [5]. For older adults, identifying behavioral health and mental health resources is very important. Adequate social and emotional support is associated with reduced risks of mental illness, physical illness, and mortality [5]. Adults aged 65 or older are more likely than adults aged 50–64 to report that they rarely or never receive the social and emotional support they need [5]. Additionally, adult males aged 50 or older are more likely than women to report that they rarely or never receive the emotional support they need [5].

The term *behavioral health* is frequently in use today. It is viewed as a less stigmatizing label than the term mental health. Behavioral health emphasizes the importance of mental health and also promotes health and wellness behaviors [6]. Health and wellness behaviors include endeavors that older clients can engage in that could improve their mental health, emotional health, or behavioral health. Behavioral health interventions include but are not limited to psychiatry, counseling services, psychotherapy, and behavior analysis. Counseling and psychotherapy is often not a preferred option for individuals aging in place and requiring home healthcare. Counseling and psychotherapy benefits are often minimized by caregivers who may be more focused on the older patient's physical health and well-being. This realism exists despite research findings that show that older adults often prefer psychotherapy to pharmacological interventions. Some counseling and psychotherapy models have proven to be quite effective with this population. Frequently used interventions include cognitive behavioral therapy, problem solving therapy, interpersonal therapy, and life review or reminiscence therapy [7]. These therapies are known to assist older adults in adjusting to their current circumstances, continuing to find meaning in life, and remaining flexible regarding expectations of self, the world, and others. These therapies can also aid older clients in remembering positive experiences from their past. Overall counseling and psychotherapy services assist older patients in managing anxiety and depression symptoms and developing coping skills and can improve their perceived overall quality of life.

Other non-pharmacological interventions (NPIs) include family therapy, geriatric group therapy, laughter therapy, art therapy, music therapy, animal-assisted therapy, and general behavior management [8–10]. Additionally, applied behavior analysts apply techniques that target behavioral health concerns by focusing on the functionality of behaviors and environmental factors. Behavior analysts work with older patients and their families to address behavior concerns. Studies suggest exercise as a favorable option for mild to moderate depression. However, those with physical limitations may be restricted in their participation [7]. Nonetheless, there is emphasis on older patients remaining as active as possible. Physical activity is often included as part of a patient's behavior plan in order to enhance mood. Geriatric mental health therapy, which focuses on the behavioral health needs of individuals over 60, is a growing discipline, yet more professionals are needed to support the behavioral health demands of this rapidly growing population. Research shows that nearly one out of five older Americans presented with at least one mental health disorder [11]. There is a dire need for high-quality mental health services that will effectively address the psychosocial needs of individuals in late life [12]. Additionally, these services can be beneficial to caregivers as they strive to manage the behavioral, emotional, and mental health symptoms displayed by older adults.

Behavioral Healthcare: Natural Environment Versus Office Setting

When providing behavioral health interventions to the older adults, the home milieu presents a more trustworthy environment. Comfort levels are maximized due to familiar surroundings, and rapport building is less of a trial. Clients are generally appreciative of providers' efforts to get to know them on their turf. Moreover, the natural environment generates opportunities for building therapeutic alliances with family and significant others. Stressors such as travel time, wait time, exposure to infectious diseases, disruptions in routine, and caregiver burden are minimized or eliminated when supportive services are provided in the home setting. Services delivered in the home environment encourage client autonomy and control. Home-based services also generate more holistic and culturally sensitive assessments and care plans. All of these factors can positively influence behavioral health outcomes. Many older adults grew up in a time when mental illness was stigmatized and when all forms of psychological distress were written off as aging or quickly diagnosed as dementia. Today, many are partaking in counseling or therapy and are reaping the benefits. Many are also exploring issues unrelated to aging through behavior intervention services [10].

Behavioral health conditions such as depression, anxiety, and psychosis are often identified in the primary care setting. Many primary care practices offer behavioral health screenings, with these screenings routinely occurring prior to contacts with primary care physicians, physician assistants, or nurse practitioners [12]. The addition of behavioral health services in the primary care setting promotes interprofessionalism and more positive outcomes for older patients. Subsequent home interventions are often extensions of primary medical care. The integration of primary medical care with behavioral health is viewed as an innovative, best practice approach to the provision of care for aging persons of the world [6]. Research in recent years has revealed the benefits of primary care and behavioral healthcare (PCHC) integration. This integration improves treatment outcomes, promotes patient independence and patient satisfaction, and focuses providers' attention on psychological, social, and mental health and substance-related factors that may be linked to medical outcomes [6].

Two major behavioral health conditions affecting older adults include late life depression and dementia. The National Institute of Mental Health does not define dementia as a mental illness but as a neurological (medical) disorder defined by loss of cognitive functioning. Nonetheless, mental health and behavioral health interventions are beneficial to patients with both conditions due to significant parallels between the two conditions. Very often, depression and dementia are experienced by the older adult at the same time. Researchers have posited that decreases in executive function, cognitive inhibition, cognitive control, memory, and concentration are symptoms of pseudodementia [13]. Behavioral and psychological symptoms of dementia include depression, agitation, aggression, apathy, irritability, disinhibition, disruptive behaviors, and psychotic symptoms [14]. According to the research literature, the risk of developing dementia is 28% higher in persons with mild cognitive impairment and patients who have depressive symptoms [15].

Pharmacological interventions (PIs) are also used to treat behavioral health conditions. Selective serotonin reuptake inhibitors (SSRIs) are pharmacological interventions (PIs) frequently used to treat depression, anxiety, and other psychological conditions in older patients. Research findings have revealed that SSRIs have less adverse reactions and side effects. Electroconvulsive therapy (ECT) is still recognized in the psychiatric and medical community as being the most effective treatment for severe depression accompanied by psychosis. Yet, many still view the inducement of seizure activity in the brain to be an extreme and unsafe option for older adults. There has been more research conducted on pharmacological treatments with these findings tending to support pharmacological interventions as the preferred course of treatment. However, many research scholars and clinicians are advocating for more clinical trials on non-pharmacological interventions (NPIs) to determine their influence on person-centered, quality of life, and well-being outcomes [7, 15].

Certain life experiences may place individuals who are older at risk for depression. These life experiences may include relocating to a new residence, acquiring a disability or chronic medical condition, losing a spouse to death, or experiencing a loss of dignity and independence. Misuse or abuse of prescribed or addictive substances can intensify depressive symptoms. The occurrence of depressive symptoms tends to increase with age; however, depression is not considered a typical part of aging. Depression is treatable in 80% of cases. In-home behavioral health providers can work with the client (and family, if applicable) to address life experiences that place the client at risk for depression [16]. Researchers discussed the role happiness plays in the health of individuals who are older. Happiness is self-defined and requires a high level of self-awareness [17]. Happiness domains comprise the physical, psychological, social, economic, religious, and spiritual aspects of the individual [17]. Individuals with high spirituality experience low levels of death anxiety. Individuals experiencing death anxiety often experience a diminished sense of well-being, sensitivity to death and dying issues, poorer cognitive status, a perception of having less control over life, and poor mental health in general [18]. Spirituality increases hope, optimism, resiliency, task orientation, and sense of control [19]. Additionally, social support, maintaining a positive perception, and good family relations positively correlate with higher levels of health. Social support and life satisfaction are central to behavioral health. Social supports are emotional, informational, and instrumental [20, 21]. Life satisfaction is influenced by socioeconomics, health, and environmental factors. Many of the aforementioned facets can moderate the prevalence of mental conditions such as depression [22].

Community-Based Programs

The Centers for Disease Control and the National Association of Chronic Disease Directors increased awareness of how depression can be effectively addressed through community-based programs. In the *State of Mental Health and Aging in America Issue Brief 2: The State of Mental Health and Aging in America*, they introduced three evidence-based programs that have been successfully replicated [24–27]. These programs are still impacting communities of older persons in 2023. Details about these three programs and others can be found in Table 8.1. Critical elements of these programs include symptom identification, continuous assessment, evidence-based interventions, and regular reviews and treatment adjustments. These community-based programs have aided individuals who experience depression and other psychological conditions in later life. Home care has been described as a "medical home" due to its reliance on team-based functions. Programs such as IMPACT and PROSPECTS have been highlighted as examples of integrated care interventions targeting mental health and substance use in older adults [12, 24]. Community-based mental health programs can prevent institutionalization or placement in a more restrictive setting. With convenient support, patients who are older are able to reside in their homes and communities with a greater sense of dignity, regardless of financial standing or ability level. Community-based mental health programs for older adults target diverse symptomatology. Given our aging society, an increase in such programs, globally, would be beneficial.

Table 8.1 Community-based programs [23–26]

Program name	Descriptive summary	Outcomes
Healthy IDEAS	Designed to detect and manage depressive symptoms among at-risk older adults and their caregivers through existing community-based case management services. The program is delivered by nonmental health professionals, such as case managers, social workers, and care coordinators, who employ a short-term, focused intervention to support better management of depressive symptoms and increased engagement in meaningful activities. Healthy IDEAS engages local mental health experts (coaches) to provide backup and support for staff	Fewer symptoms of depression Decreased physical pain Better ability to recognize and self-treat symptoms Improved well-being through achievement of personal goals Healthy IDEAS is a national model with measurable results and demonstrated benefits for older adults, service providers, and community mental/behavioral health practitioners. The pilot study and large-scale demonstration of healthy IDEAS were conducted in Houston, Texas, as part of a community-academic partnership managed by Care for Elders in collaboration with Baylor College of Medicine
PEARLS (Program to Encourage Active, Rewarding Lives)	PEARLS (Program to Encourage Active, Rewarding Lives) is a treatment program designed to reduce symptoms of depression and improve quality of life among older adults. More than 50 sites in 18 states use PEARLS, with more organizations enrolling each year. The program consists of six to eight in-home counseling sessions that focus on the following goals: Solving problems, becoming socially and physically active, scheduling enjoyable activities	A University of Washington study determined that PEARLS participants had a 50% or higher reduction in symptoms of depression, and 36% showed complete remission. The participants' quality of life, both physical and emotional, also improved, resulting in fewer hospitalizations. Later studies showed that the program is also effective for adults of all ages with epilepsy
IMPACT Care or IMPACT Model (Improving Mood: Providing Access to Collaborative Treatment) or Collaborative Care Model (CoCM)	The IMPACT model is recognized as effective treatment for a wide range of behavioral health disorders – Not just depression. A team-based collaborative care approach addresses anxiety and trauma disorders, chronic pain, substance use disorders including alcohol and opioids, and ADHD	Collaborative care more than doubled the effectiveness of depression treatment for older adults in primary care settings. At 12 months, about half of the patients receiving collaborative care reported at least a 50% reduction in depressive symptoms, compared with only 19% of those in usual care
Prevention of Suicide in Primary Care Elderly: Collaborative Trial (PROSPECT)	PROSPECT aims to prevent suicide among older primary care patients by reducing suicidal ideation and depression. It also aims to reduce their risk of death. The intervention components are (1) recognition of depression and suicidal ideation by primary care physicians, (2) application of a treatment algorithm for geriatric depression in the primary care setting, and (3) treatment management by health specialists (e.g., nurses, social workers, psychologists)	The treatment algorithm assists primary care physicians in making appropriate care choices during the acute, continuation, and maintenance phases of treatment. Health specialists collaborate with physicians to monitor patients and encourage patient adherence to recommended treatments. Patients are treated and monitored for 24 months for depressive symptomatology and suicidality
PATH	PATH is a 12-week home-delivered intervention that focuses on the patients' ecosystem (i.e., the patient, the caregiver, and the home environment). The goals of PATH are to reduce patients' depression and disability by facilitating problem solving and adaptive functioning	Preliminary study findings suggest that PATH is well accepted and efficacious in depressed elders with major depression, cognitive impairment, and disability

Using the Home Environment to Accentuate Traditional Assessment Procedures

In regard to the population of older adults, the home environment is the ideal setting to conduct behavioral health and mental capacity assessments. It goes without saying that the home environment "speaks volumes" and transcends the traditional assessment setting. Behavioral health providers are able to understand more fully the influences of behavioral health on various life domains (e.g., physical health, emotional well-being, family dynamics, intimacy, spirituality, safety, and community), as well as the impact of these domains on behavioral health. Home-based assessments are more accurate, comprehensive, and culturally sensitive. They afford opportunities to consider the client in the context of the home and community. Also, visible and shared artifacts can be incorporated into the assessment process, as well as observations from family, friends, and neighbors.

Conducting assessments in the home allows the behavioral health provider to discern various points of intersectionality within the home ecological system and to use this understanding as a framework for interprofessional collaboration. Similarly, the client's mood, thought processes, and levels of compliance and motivation can *intersect* with the treatment agendas of interprofessional team members. Thus, behavioral health professionals can be an asset to the team by providing guidance on strategies that can increase patient engagement and compliance. For the behavioral health professional, fundamental competencies such as building rapport, establishing a therapeutic alliance, asking relevant (respectful) questions, and demonstrating critical observation skills create a basis for conducting quality assessments. Table 8.2 portrays diagnostic instruments that can be used to assess the behavioral health of clients who are older. While assessments are vitally important to the behavioral health process, they should not be executed without client approval. Clients must be educated on both the benefits and risks of assessment procedures. Consent should be obtained prior to involving the client in any formal assessment procedures. Additionally, engaging in an open discussion about the purpose of the assessment tool, how it will be used, and who will have access to the results is important. The conscientious, intentional behavioral health professional should never attempt to use an assessment tool without proper credentialing or training nor without proper written and oral consent.

Early detection of behavioral health conditions is very important. Sadly, depression in late life often goes undetected and untreated [7]. Thus, concerted efforts must be directed toward employing instruments that can be effective in identifying behavioral health needs. Table 8.2 provides information on commonly used diagnostic instruments [12]. The conscientious behavioral healthcare provider, if not skilled in the administration of specific diagnostic tools, must at least be familiar with the purpose of the instruments. The diagnostic assessment marks the beginning of the behavior health treatment process. It involves the gathering of information for

Table 8.2 Types of diagnostic instruments [12]

Prescreening diagnostics	Depression	Anxiety	Cognitive	Physical functioning and caregiver burden	Other
Comprehensive Composite International Diagnostic Interview 65 plus (CIDI65+)	Geriatric Depression Scale (GDS) (long and short version) (GDS-30 GDS-15)	Panic Frequency Questionnaire (PFQ)	Montreal Cognitive Assessment (MoCA)	Functional Activities Questionnaire (FAQ)	Epworth Sleepiness Scale (ESS)
Questionnaire for Assessing the Impact of the COVID-19 Pandemic in Older Adults (QAICPOA)	Cornell Scale for Depression in Dementia (CSDD)	Beck Anxiety Inventory-Primary Care (BAI)	Mini-Mental Status Exam (MMSE)	Caregiver Assessment of Function and Upset (CAFU)	Activities of Daily Living Prevention Instrument (ADL-PI)
The Neuropsychiatry Inventory (NPI)	Hamilton Depression Rating Scale (HDRS)		The 7 Min Cognitive Screen (Mini-Cog)	Lawton Instrumental Activities of Daily Living Scale (IADL)	Pittsburgh Sleep Quality Index (PSQI)
Composite International Diagnostic Interview-Primary Care (CIDI-PC)	Beck Depression Inventory (BDI) Beck Depression Inventory-Primary Care (BDI-PC)			Activities of Daily Living Scale (ADLs)	Alcohol Use Disorders Identification Test (AUDIT)
Test Quality of Life Inventory (QoLI)	Center for Epidemiologic Studies Depression Scale (CESD-20)			Zarit Caregiver Burden Interview (ZBI)	Survey of Activities and Fear of Falling in the Elderly (SAFE)

the purpose of diagnosing mental health conditions, distinguishing between mental and physical health conditions, and assessing coping capacity in various life domains. Assessment results can influence care planning and decision-making of other interprofessional team members.

Safety Considerations and Crisis Planning

Individuals in late life often experience apprehension about their emotional and physical safety. Safety is defined as the condition of being protected from danger, risk, or injury. Definitions of crisis planning typically address procedures for addressing sudden or emergency situations. Behavioral health providers must never underestimate the nexus between behavioral health and emotional and physical safety. Early in the therapeutic relationship, there should be gentle conversations

Table 8.3 Fear and concerns about safety

(Psychological/internal)	(Physical/external)
Loss of independence	Loss of accessibility
Vulnerability to harm, abuse, or exploitation	Loss of mobility
Powerlessness	Hearing loss
Death	Other sensory deficits
Being alone	Loss of function
Guilt pertaining to caregiver burden	Falling in isolation
Loss of dignity and independence	Falling and getting hurt
Memory loss or cognitive decline	Frailty
Loss of privacy	Being trapped (fires, natural disasters, etc.)
Loss of friends, social status	Robbery and break-ins
Lack of meaning and purpose	Overmedicated or substance dependency
Loss of mental resilience	Equipment, devices, or alarms not working

about fears and concerns as they relate to safety and well-being. These should not be minimized but validated as legitimate. Table 8.3 depicts common fears and concerns about safety that older clients might have. These aspects if not addressed or diminished can have significant impact on the health and wellness of older clients. Safety and crisis planning should incorporate the fears and concerns of clients as well as the observations of family members and caregivers. It is important to communicate to clients that many of their fears and concerns are typical during late life, and can be managed with support and guidance. Behavioral health professionals working with clients who are older must be proficient in assessing suicidality, psychosis, substance use, disordered eating, and other conditions that might threaten safety or result in a crisis. Family members must be supported in understanding these conditions and responding appropriately. It is important that behavioral health professionals work closely with other interprofessional team members to address issues pertaining to safety, crisis prevention, and crisis management.

Interprofessional Collaboration and Referrals

Upon receipt of a referral, the conscientious behavioral health professional, regardless of discipline (i.e., psychology, psychiatry, clinical mental health, rehabilitation counseling, social work, marriage and family therapy), should ask the referral source about other providers who are involved in the patient's care, particularly those providing home-based care. Prompt written and verbal consent should be given by the client for ongoing consultations with all interprofessional team members. Behavioral health providers must be knowledgeable of community resources and referral protocols. The behavioral health professional must be committed to sharing relevant resources and educating interprofessional team members about specific treatments being delivered within the home setting. These consultations and information sharing events may not always be "billable," but these professional exchanges are considered accountable (and quality) care practices. Concerns relating to a colleague's practice decisions should be handled directly and transparently, with the goal being to maximize client outcomes via respectful interprofessional collaborations.

Tele-Behavioral Health Services

Tele-behavioral health services are beneficial in the same vein as traditional home-based services. Principally, these real-time, face-to-face services comprise a convenient and compassionate mode of service delivery. Issues pertaining to mobility and travel and transportation are minimized, as well as worries about infectious diseases. Currently, the Centers for Medicare and Medicaid Services (CMS) authorizes payments for behavioral health services to a select number of disciplines. This payment disparity is beyond the scope of this chapter. However, we are pleased at the ongoing advocacy aimed at eliminating this disparity given the demand for increased behavioral health services for individuals who are older. When it comes to the provision of tele-behavioral health services, it is imperative that providers engage in regular reviews of the code of ethics for their discipline. They should also review (extensively) the standards and regulations set forth by their licensing or certifying board or commission. Most ethical codes and state or national licensing or certifying boards mandate proficiency or compliance in the following areas:

(a) HIPAA compliance and secure audio- and videoconferencing technology.
(b) Encryption standards that meet applicable legal requirements.
(c) Informed consent and user orientation to tele-services to include a discussion of the risks, benefits, and responsibilities associated with technology-assisted services.
(d) Documentation of provider training on ethically engaging clients in tele-behavioral health services.
(e) Assuring that technologically assisted services are appropriate for clients given their intellectual, emotional, cognitive, linguistic, and functional needs.
(f) Practicing within allowed jurisdictions.
(g) Emergency procedures for when provider is not available.
(h) Technology failures and interruptions.
(i) Verification steps to ensure client identity at the beginning and various points throughout the episodes of telecare [27].

Clients should be given a choice regarding participation in tele-services. If they are more comfortable with face-to-face in-person interventions, their preference should be respected. The conscientious behavioral health provider's treatment decisions are always based on what is best and most comfortable for the client. Providers should forewarn clients about the possibility of communication errors occurring due to a lack of visual cues, poor lighting, poor connectivity, or voice intonations. It is also imperative that professionals ensure that clients have access to and understand how to effectively utilize their Internet and electronic devices.

Tool Box: Behavioral Health Activities for Use with Older Clients

Table 8.4 introduces a few behavioral health activities that can be used with older adults in the home setting. These therapeutic activities can be used to address a range of emotive states stemming from body image changes due to aging, physical illness and disability, loneliness, cognitive decline, or bereavement. The objective of each therapeutic activity is provided. Many of these activities and aims were developed by the authors. This chapter concludes with an example of how behavioral health professionals can collaborate with other interprofessional team members. The collaboration is based on the Case Study: Jeralean.

Case Study: IP Collaboration on Behalf of Jeralean

As mentioned previously, the behavioral health provider must secure written consent from the client before collaborating with members of the interprofessional team. In the case study of Jeralean, the behavioral health professional would demonstrate interprofessional collaboration by implementing the following steps:

1. Upon receipt of client consent, compose and deliver an introductory email or phone call to each of the interprofessional team members, summarizing behavioral health treatment goals and activities and requesting a prompt phone call if certain maladaptive emotions or behaviors are observed.
2. Obtain a schedule of when team members will be visiting the client in order to avoid schedule conflicts.
3. Keep the referral source abreast of client progress (on a need-to-know basis).
4. Consult with the dietician about simple and healthy meal preparation and about foods that will enhance energy, memory, and sleep.
5. Consult with the occupational therapist about exercises and rehabilitation techniques that can be incorporated into the behavioral health sessions, particularly for activities requiring movement and fine motor coordination.
6. Consult with the physical therapist about exercise prescriptions and approved exercises and physical activities.
7. Consult with the prosthetist about factors influencing poor use of prosthesis, as well as common concerns about body image.
8. Consult with the social worker about resources for the installation of cost-effective home modifications and about social and leisure organizations that may be of interest to both Jeralean and Alice.
9. Lastly, the behavioral health provider should offer both mom and daughter the opportunity to participate in family counseling.

Table 8.4 Behavior health tool box

Activity	Aim
Guided imagery and relaxation	To assist with emotional self-regulation, to reduce anxiety and promote a sense of wellness
Grief and loss	To provide education and support for coping with grief and loss
Mirror Mirror!	To assist with the psychosocial adjustment (adaptation) to aging to include body image issues
Watch it grow	To encourage gardening in the yard or aboveground, to instill hope and purpose
Let's dance!	To provide therapy via movement and music, to reduce anxiety and depression
Laughter is the best medicine	To encourage humor and spontaneity
Getting over the hump	To visualize and identify barriers to life, health, and happiness
Remember when	To guide clients in recapturing memories and putting them in proper perspective
Memory timeline	To aid clients in putting their life in perspective by revisiting milestones
Memory cues	To identify and encourage use of memory prompts and aids
Artwork	To promote relaxation and a sense of purpose
I am in control (of my fears and concerns)	To help clients resolve fears and concerns, self-empowerment
Scrapbooking	To promote relaxation and a sense of purpose and accomplishment
Journaling (audio)	To promote memory and to create a legacy artifact for loved ones
Look what I did today	To promote a sense of joy, purpose, and accomplishment
Who am I? (now and then)	To promote a sense of pride, accomplishment, self-acceptance, and self-efficacy

Chapter Summary

The term behavioral health in many instances is used instead of more stigmatizing terms. Behavioral health services for older patients often include counseling, psychotherapy, psychiatry, and behavior analysis. These services are vital in meeting the behavioral, emotional, and/or mental health needs of older clients or patients. In many instances, the home environment is the ideal setting for behavioral health interventions. As discussed in this chapter, many older adults are good candidates for these interventions; yet, behavioral health interventions are often a last (care) resort. Behavioral health interventions can benefit family members and caregivers. Behavioral health providers can be great contributors to interprofessional teams.

Discussion Questions

1. What are common causes of mental illness or psychological distress in older adults?
2. Give a specific example of an opportunity for a behavioral health professional to collaborate with an interprofessional team member.

Multiple Choice Questions

1. Behavioral health emphasizes the importance of mental health but also promotes (select the *best* answer).
   (a) Financial literacy and stability
   (b) Coping and adjustment
   (c) Health and wellness
   (d) Community engagement
2. Examples of behavioral health professionals include
   (a) Nutritionists
   (b) Geriatric counselors
   (c) Psychiatrists
   (d) B and C
3. In primary care settings, behavioral health screenings are typically conducted.
   (a) Over the telephone when the initial appointment is made
   (b) During the initial appointment paperwork
   (c) At the conclusion of the medical appointment
   (d) Prior to contact with physicians, physician assistants, or nurse practitioner
4. Which of the following are appropriate behavioral health activities to use with clients who are older?
   (a) Activities focusing on estate planning
   (b) Activities focusing on memory loss
   (c) Activities focusing on grief and loss
   (d) B and C
5. Which of the following is a scale most commonly used to diagnose anxiety?
   (a) Panic Frequently Questionnaire
   (b) Mini-Mental Status Exam
   (c) Lawton Instrumental Activities of Daily Living Scale
   (d) Beck Depression Inventory

References

1. Older Adults Living With Serious Mental Illness The State of the Behavioral Health Workforce – Substance Abuse and Mental Health Services Administration 2019 Older Adults Living with Serious Mental Illness The State of the Behavioral Health Workforce (samhsa.gov)
2. Administration on Aging, Administration for Community Living. (2018). *2017 profile of older Americans*. U.S. Department of Health and Human Services.
3. U.S. Census Bureau. (2017). The nation's older population is still growing: The nation's population is becoming more diverse. Release Number, CB17–100.
4. Shahboulaghi, M., Moghaddam, A. G., & Khoshnou, H. (2017). Mental health in the elderly and its predictive factors. *World Family Medicine Journal: Incorporating the Middle East Journal of Family Medicine, 99*(5588), 1–8.
5. Centers for Disease Control and Prevention and National Association of Chronic Disease Directors. (2008). *The state of mental health and aging in America issue brief 1: What do the data tell us?* National Association of Chronic Disease Directors.
6. Hills, W. (2019). Behavioral health and new models of service delivery for an aging world: Public/private partnerships to develop best practices of care for older adults. *Medical Science Pulse, 13*, 13–29.
7. Mikesell, L. (2021). *Mental health interventions for the elderly*. Older Age Psychiatry.
8. Reinhardt, M. M., & Cohen, C. I. (2015). Late-life psychosis: Diagnosis and treatment. *Current Psychiatry Reports, 17*, 1. https://doi.org/10.1007/s11920-014-0542-0
9. Abraha, I., Rimland, J. M., Trotta, F. M., Dell'Aquila, G., Cruz-Jentoft, A., Petrovic, M., et al. (2017). Systematic review of systematic reviews of non-pharmacological interventions to treat behavioral disturbances in older patients with dementia. The SENATOR-OnTop series. *BMJ Open, 7*(3), e012759.
10. https://www.goodtherapy.org/learn-about-therapy/issues/aging (11/21/19).
11. Institute of Medicine. (2012). The mental health and substance use workforce for older adults: In *Whose hands*? National Academies Press.
12. Hyer, L. (2013). *Psychological treatment of older adults: A holistic model*. Springer Publishing Company.
13. Valiengo, L. D. C. L., Stella, F., & Forlenza, O. V. (2016). Mood disorders in the elderly: Prevalence, functional impact, and management challenges. *Neuropsychiatric Disease and Treatment, 12*, 2105–2114.
14. Ropacki, S. A., & Jeste, D. V. (2005). Epidemiology of and risk factors for psychosis of Alzheimer's disease: A review of 55 studies published from 1990 to 2003. *American Journal of Psychiatry, 162*(11), 2022–2030.
15. Rodakowski, J., & Skidmore, E. R. (2017). Non-pharmacological interventions for early cognitive decline. *American Journal of Gerontology, 37*(5), 665–676.
16. Chapman, D. P., Perry, G. S., & Strine, T. W. (2005). The vital link between chronic disease and depressive disorders. *Preventing Chronic Disease, 2*(1), A14.
17. Sharmila, K. (2020). Role of happiness in health of elderly. *Indian Journal of Gerontology, 34*(4).
18. Sharma, P., Asthana, H. S., Gambhir, I. S., & Ranjan, J. K. (2019). Death anxiety among elderly people: Role of gender, spirituality and mental health. *Indian Journal of Gerontology, 33*(3).
19. Zimmer, Z., Jagger, C., Chiu, C. T., Ofstedal, M. B., & Rojo, F. (2016). Spirituality, religiosity, aging and health in global perspective: A review. *SSM Popul Health, 2*, 373–381.
20. Strine, T. W., Chapman, D. P., Balluz, L., & Mokdad, A. H. (2008). Health-related quality of life and health behaviors by social and emotional support: Their relevance to psychiatry and medicine. *Social Psychiatry and Psychiatric Epidemiology, 43*, 151–159.
21. Strine, T. W., Chapman, D. P., Balluz, L., Moriarty, D. G., & Mokdad, A. H. (2008). The associations between life satisfaction and health-related quality of life, chronic illness, and health behaviors among U.S. community-dwelling adults. *Journal of Community Health, 33*, 40–50.

22. Linton, S. J., & Nordin, E. (2016). A 5-year follow-up evaluation of the health and economic consequences of an early cognitive behavioural intervention for back pain: A randomized, controlled trial. *Spine, 31*, 853–858.
23. Centers for Disease Control and Prevention and National Association of Chronic Disease Directors. (2009). *The state of mental health and aging in America issue brief 2: Addressing depression in older adults: Selected evidence-based programs.* National Association of Chronic Disease Directors.
24. Healthy IDEAS Programs. (2017). National Center for Chronic Disease Prevention and Health Promotion, Division of Population Health (2018); Advancing Integrated Mental Health Solution, University of Washington (2022) https://healthyideasprograms.org/
25. National Center for Chronic Disease Prevention and Health Promotion, Division of Population Health. (2018). *PEARLS.* https://www.cdc.gov/prc/resources/tools/pearls.html#:~:text=PEARLS%20(Program%20to%20Encourage%20Active,all%2Dage%20adults%20with%20epilepsy.&text=More%20than%2050%20sites%20in,more%20organizations%20enrolling%20each%20year.
26. Impact: Improving mood, promoting access to collaborative treatment (2023). *The University of Washington, Psychiatry and Behavioral Sciences, Division of Population Health.* http://aims.uw.edu/impact-improving-mood-promoting-access-collaborative-treatment
27. Codes of Ethics on TeleMental Health, E-Therapy, Digital Ethics, and Social Media, by Ofer Zur, Ph.D. (2022). https://www.zurinstitute.com/resources/ethics-of-telehealth/

Chapter 9
Other Relevant Home Care Services: Prosthetics and Orthotics, Pharmacy Services, Durable Medical Equipment, and Nutritional Services

Scott Bretl, Adan Vazquez, and Geordan Stapleton

Learning Objectives
1. Summarize differences in prosthetic and orthotic care for older patients.
2. Identify benefits and risks in prosthetic and orthotic care when working with patients who are older.
3. Understand and address potential obstacles when working with patients who are older who might use prosthetic and/or orthotic devices.
4. Articulate examples of durable medical equipment utilized in the home care setting.
5. Articulate examples of nutritional concerns associated with older patients.
6. Describe the role of pharmacological services when caring for older patients.

Introduction to Prosthetics and Orthotics

The prosthetist-orthotist has become an increasingly important healthcare specialist in the lives of the older patient population, and the requirements of their work result in unique challenges to providing optimal treatment in the home environment. As a

Supplementary Information The online version contains supplementary material available at https://doi.org/10.1007/978-3-031-40889-2_9.

S. Bretl (✉) · A. Vazquez
Department of Prosthetics and Orthotics, College of Health Sciences, Alabama State University, Montgomery, AL, USA
e-mail: sbretl@alasu.edu; avazquez@alasu.edu

G. Stapleton
Performance Nutrition Division, New York Mets, Port St. Lucie, FL, USA
e-mail: Gstapleton@nymets.com

D. H. Stapleton, S. Bossie (eds.), *Home Care for Older Adults Using Interprofessional Teams*, https://doi.org/10.1007/978-3-031-40889-2_9

prosthetist, the clinical professional provides care to patients with partial or total absence of limbs by designing, fabricating, and fitting prostheses – or artificial limbs. Orthotists work with those presenting with neuromuscular or musculoskeletal impairments by designing, fabricating, and fitting orthoses – or braces. Often dually trained, these members of the allied healthcare team develop treatment plans to address functional limitation and disability. Though they direct the creation, use, and maintenance of medical devices, their services are centered around the patient and his or her changing needs longitudinally. The prosthetist-orthotist is constantly teaching, evaluating, and adjusting such that the prosthetic or orthotic "tool" can maximally support regained function and mobility.

The increasing prevalence of dysvascular conditions in this country has resulted in 66% of a prosthetist's patients having undergone limb amputation as a result of disease processes, and 37% of patients are aged 65 years or older. While amputation-related conditions of diabetes and peripheral vascular disease are alarmingly associated with increased mortality of the older patient, the movement disorders associated with orthotic treatment typically carry a lower mortality. Comparatively, 44% of an orthotist's patients require bracing as a result of disease processes, and 27% are 65 or older [1]. In countries like the USA, older individuals comprise nearly half the burden of disease [2]. For both the prosthetic and orthotic categories of body impairment, a patient's independence, their mobility, and the health of their remaining anatomy can be greatly impacted in a negative way without intervention, so the follow-through of prosthetic or orthotic care is of the utmost importance.

For a subset of the average prosthetic and orthotic patient population, completion of the treatment process can be disrupted due to various needs and challenges of the patient. Topmost on the list for many is transportation, and all the logistical details involved in getting a mobility-challenged individual from their home to the clinic. Patients on a prosthetist-orthotist's caseload may not currently drive a vehicle (or may never have driven a vehicle) and may be utilizing one of many versions of an assistive device. A full evaluation may uncover that they are notably limited in their community mobility with concerns for safety, and yet a traditional clinical office visit requires the traversing of many elements of the community environment. Older patients are more likely to shoulder these challenges, and in some areas, outpatient clinics deal with related "no-call, no-shows" and canceled or rescheduled appointments on a daily basis. As such, a consideration to instead treat the patient in their home has both the best interests of the patient and the best interests of the organization in mind.

In the case of treatment and services in the home environment, the clinical practitioner must decide what typical or traditional treatment processes require modification for the varying living environments. Though it can be a significant challenge to bring the clinic to the patient in this way, services in the home offer a unique opportunity to witness activities of daily living (ADLs) in real time and as they are meant to occur, to allow the prosthetist-orthotist to pick up on the nuances of patient needs.

This population may already be dealing with issues of agism, multimorbidity, inadequate income security, and more [2]. In recent years, insurance limitations have plagued access to prosthetic and orthotic care, made worse by the population of prosthetist-orthotists that is not growing fast enough to meet the health needs of those entering retirement age [3, 4]. In the case of prosthetics, due to a relatively decreased activity level compared to other adults, geriatric patients are often prevented from receiving higher-end components that have advanced safety features. In this way, there are limited geriatric specific components and device options that are routinely eligible for insurance payment – likely due to a lack of geriatric representation in prosthetic studies [4]. With many challenges, it is important that the practitioner and his or her organization consider those aspects within their power to change, in order to seek improved outcomes for their patients at risk. Though not without its own considerations and challenges, an adjustment to the location of care and services may be at the top of that list. This is all without mentioning a general preference for patients at this age to remain in familiar surroundings for their care.

Natural Environment Versus Traditional Setting

The needs of the prosthetist-orthotist – and the older patient – vary throughout the treatment plan, depending upon the stage of care. In the traditional setting, when a physician prescription has been provided, services begin with thorough patient evaluation, with the practitioner making note of subjective and objective qualities of the patient and his or her condition. Following the International Classification of Functioning, Disability and Health (ICF) biopsychosocial model, prosthetist-orthotists often approach patient evaluations recognizing the multidimensionality of the concepts of function and disability [5]. They aim to uncover details of a patient's body function and structure (and impairments thereof), a patient's activities specific to tasks or actions (and limitations thereof), a patient's participation broader to life situations (and restrictions thereof), and environmental and personal factors that may serve as either facilitators or barriers to successful rehabilitation. A patient's quality of life is believed to largely be a function of these details [5]. The patient evaluation then involves interview and measurement – informing a treatment plan with patient-stated facts, practitioner-observed qualities, and concretely measured quantities, as well as more abstract characterizations of presentation.

The appointment environment makes little difference for subjective aspects of the evaluation session that collect information via conversation or question-answer, and in some ways a setting in the natural environment provides the prosthetist-orthotist with more unfiltered observations relevant to treatment decisions – as in the case of details around a patient's attention, cognition, emotion, motivation, or self-care. In P&O, relevant objective assessment involves use of various physical measurement tools as well as appropriate furniture and space for body positioning and clinical observation of a patient both standing and walking. Not to be ignored is the importance of attention to a clinician's own body mechanics while managing the evaluation stage of care in the home setting. Services may need to be provided without practitioner stools or patient beds with height adjustability, and even a safe chair with weight-bearing-capable armrests may not be found among the household furnishings. Still, the prosthetist-orthotist can easily adapt their services with appropriate communication of expectations with the patient. This is, after all, not unlike the practitioner who makes on-call visits to the hospital or routinely sees patients in a skilled nursing facility.

The selection of treatment goals and outcome measurement tools to assess progress toward those goals is perhaps a simpler task in working with the older patient at home; details about the patient's living environment and depictions of a-day-in-the-life-of-the-patient are directly observable in real time, giving higher likelihood to goals and measures that are relevant and specific [6]. Most healthcare disciplines realize similar benefits of working with the patient in the natural environment [7].

A new evaluation of the patient often concludes with a prosthetic or orthotic prescriptive recommendation, with the prosthetist-orthotist using clinical judgment and expertise, patient input, and supporting evidence from academic literature to justify a device design that would support improved function and independence while also meeting an insurance provider's requirements for medical necessity and policy coverage [8]. Device selections may include prefabricated options – off-the-shelf solutions that are sized-to-fit and partially adjustable – or fully custom devices that are built uniquely for one patient and their anatomy.

Orthotists range in their use of different device types for their patients, partially as a function of the body segment being treated – as few as 18% of ankle-foot orthoses are prefabricated, while it is as much as 40% among spinal orthoses [1]. A challenge of the home setting for the orthotist may come in the consideration of how to achieve a negative impression or similar model of the body segment with minimal materials, tools, and mess. The traditional method involves plaster, fiberglass, or other synthetic casting wrap that sets prior to tooled removal; however, the use of non-plaster options is best for avoiding the dirtying of a patient's home. Similarly, increasing in use are 3D scanning hardware options that provide zero-mess and a more exact model in certain circumstances [9]. Still, the experienced orthotist will arrive prepared to select among multiple strategies based on a patient's presentation of muscle tone, their limb strength to assist in positioning for the shape capture process, etc. The overwhelming majority of prosthetic treatment plans involve custom socket shapes that require similar considerations for appointments in the home, though sized-to-fit options do exist.

The limitations of home care become apparent when the prosthetic or orthotic treatment plan has progressed to introduce the use of a new external device, either custom-fabricated or purchased prefabricated. Following the determination of a treatment plan, the prosthetist-orthotist oversees the fabrication or purchase process for parts or the whole of the device. These intermediate steps are comfortably handled in a traditional clinical setting, where many P&O businesses choose to maintain some amount of laboratory space devoted to various steps of fabrication or assembly. This business model exists based on the consideration of many of the daily requirements in that process. A traditional plaster cast for a custom device requires "modification" or "rectification" from its original shape (the addition or removal of plaster) to strategically influence the shaping of the final product. The process of achieving a final custom product often involves the "thermoforming" process whereby heat-moldable plastic is brought to formable temperature inside a large oven and then subjected to negative vacuum pressure as it is formed over a plaster or similar mold. Material cutting and removal tools and a sanding machine are typically requirements to turn the molded material into a finished product that is safe for patient use, and final assembly often requires the use of adhesives and rivets, among other things. Even the purchase of prefabricated parts or products requires a clinical home-base that manages shipping and receiving. While it is of little consequence to the homebound patient where exactly the fabrication or preparation process takes place, the traditional fitting process for P&O devices often relies on the convenience and availability of a lab outfitted with tools and machinery to make adjustments on-site as needed. Without this resource, the treatment process risks becoming entirely inefficient if the only solution for the clinician is to travel back and forth from a brick-and-mortar office. The need for adjustment can be a routine expectation in the fitting process and can also compromise the ability of the patient to wear a device at all.

This is, of course, not the only business model employed in the P&O space. Only 61% and 39% of prosthetic and orthotic devices, respectively, are fabricated on-site at the average P&O clinic, with the rest being outsourced to what is often referred to as a "central fabrication" facility [1]. Still, the average clinic's setup has not prioritized home health situations for older individuals. Those that have defined this as an important patient population have committed to a certain amount of "digital workflow" (e.g., CAD – computer-aided design via 3D scanning hardware and digital modification software) to minimize the need for certain materials, tools, or equipment. They have also demonstrated a commitment to convenience and efficiency with the homebound patient by outfitting vehicles with portable versions of the most essential tools and equipment, in what is often referred to as a "mobile clinic." Public health protocols throughout the COVID-19 pandemic brought attention to the advantages of this type of flexibility of care, but there is no data as of yet to point to an increasing trend. A 2022 survey of prosthetist-orthotists suggests that only 3% of direct orthotic patient care and only 6% of direct prosthetic patient care occur at the patient's residence [1]. Some businesses have instead opted to create their own transportation service to pick up and drop off patients, suggesting that this may be a financially efficient method of meeting the needs of this target population.

Follow-up care in the traditional setting often follows a rough formula for timing, perhaps unique to an individual's device type, plus many other factors. In truth, patients do not always need to be seen in predictable time intervals; though it is good for the prosthetist-orthotist to be given the opportunity to reassess a worn device for fit, function, and safety, it may be just as effective to emphasize education on problems to watch for with a new device to avoid unnecessary travel burden on the older patient. With home care, it becomes top of mind for clinicians to routinely check in with patients regarding their treatment needs to determine if the clinician's travel and time are necessary. When it is necessary, follow-up care similarly comes with the consideration of how to make needed device adjustments without a full lab facility readily nearby.

Using the Home Environment to Accentuate Traditional Assessment and Evaluation

In the assessment or evaluation for services, there are several ways in which a home setting can reinforce optimal care [10]. In traditional settings, the prosthetist-orthotist asks the patient about their current condition or function. As expected with a referral from their physician, the older patient indicates some performance limitation or barrier to independence – though the full understanding of this is reliant on the patient's ability to wholly communicate their experience. Inevitably some details of these needs are left understated, or else a crucial aspect of their daily experience is omitted altogether. Without close attention to targeted and follow-up questioning, the clinician relies too heavily on the patient knowing what is or is not important to note about their daily experience. Comparatively, in the natural home environment, a clinician is provided the golden opportunity to supplement patients' subjective descriptions with "Can you show me?" which allows the prosthetist-orthotist to identify the underlying challenge to function – and confidently develop a treatment plan which would serve to best support the routine needs in that environment. Questions about the living environment can be transformed into a tour of the patient's home with a description of activities of daily living (ADLs) in each room, and the clinician is also provided the opportunity to inform the patient of some things they could consider altering in their home environment to assist in current mobility and future mobility with a device.

In the assessment or evaluation following delivery of services, the natural environment again offers unique advantages. In the development of a treatment plan, a prosthetist-orthotist aims to provide a device that primarily balances requirements of control, comfort, cosmesis, and cost and to provide services that are timely. The success of the device in these areas may not always be apparent in the controlled clinical setting, requiring the clinician to ask the right questions of the patient or requiring the patient to provide the right details in their answers for proper assessment. In fact, numerous clinical outcome measurement surveys have been created for the P&O patient population to learn more about the patient experience in their natural environment [11, 12]. When the patient's home is the clinical setting, there exists a unique opportunity to assess the success of the device for its intended use or specifically for the situations in which the patient has the greatest need. Unique to P&O home care, the prosthetist-orthotist may use direct observations to assess whether or not the device avoids limitation in task-based activities and does so without issues such as fatigue or skin irritation, is appropriate in simplicity for the patient to independently manage and maintain, is functional with a variety of the patient's usual clothing or footwear, or is usable with low energy cost. Continuity in the care setting allows the prosthetist-orthotist to specifically evaluate function and performance with a device in the very same situations, rooms, and activities as those mentioned in the initial assessment for services.

Whether it is before or after provision of a new device, a prosthetist may advise on proper strategies and body mechanics for the patient with new lower limb amputation to manage mobility in their bed specifically or transfers to and from their chairs specifically. Instead of simply explaining how to clean and otherwise care for a new device and its components, the prosthetist may have the patient properly hand-wash their prosthetic liner interface or their suspension sleeve at their own kitchen or bathroom sink and provide direct feedback. The orthotist similarly may minimize the direct instruction of how to move an ankle-foot orthosis (AFO) between shoes and maximize the actions of the patient actually practicing it for themselves. In the event that the patient is dependent upon a caregiver, the caregiver is given the opportunity to learn the best ways to support the patient. In this way, the requirement to meet an older patient in their home becomes an opportunity for education – leaving all parties better informed in the process.

Safety Considerations and Crisis Planning

Patient safety is top of mind for the prosthetist-orthotist developing a treatment plan or assessing the current state of a patient while using a device. In fact, for most older patients, the obvious safety consideration is fall risk. Up to 70% of community-dwelling patients with chronic stroke will have fallen within the first year [13]; the fear of falling is reported among 88% of "fallers" [14], and nearly half of individuals restrict their activities because of it [15]. This risk exists among many other pathological conditions: diabetes [16], peripheral neuropathy [17], amputation [18], etc. For the prosthetist-orthotist, prominent among intrinsic factors of falling are sensory deficits, neurological/neuromuscular impairment, and musculoskeletal impairment; home conditions offer extrinsic factors that similarly enhance risk but can be largely preventable.

Custom design means that a patient's presentation of subjective qualities and objective measurements makes them either indicated or contraindicated for certain design components. For example, broadly, the older individual with balance impairment is likely indicated for an AFO, though significant fluctuations in limb volume as a result of a dialysis regimen may have the patient contraindicated for a traditional thermoplastic AFO that fully contains the posterior half of the shank. Similarly, most older patients are contraindicated for a knee-ankle-foot orthosis (KAFO) simply due to its weight and the corresponding strength of the patient's hip and knee flexors, but if it is essential that the brace crosses the knee for proper control, then the patient could be indicated for this, provided that it uses a design that reduces bulk and utilizes lightweight material. Knowledge of contraindications is often more consequential to health and safety, as in the case of an axial-loading or patellar-tendon-bearing AFO, which is contraindicated for use for those with peripheral vascular disease, knowing that the circumferential pressure risks compromising distal blood flow. In this way, the orthotist for example prioritizes patient safety in the treatment plan.

More specifically within the selection of prosthetic elements, device components are also established based on indications and contraindications. The average prosthetic device for a transtibial amputation is assembled from the combination of a type of socket, a type of interface, a type of foot, and either internal alignable componentry or a non-alignable exterior structure. Among the many combinations of design selections can be the choice of specific interfaces such as gel liner material type: thermoplastic elastomer (TPE), silicone, (poly)urethane, or proprietary "hybrid" gels. Involved in the assignment of a patient being indicated or contraindicated for one liner material (and thickness) over another are the patient's skin integrity and the desired method of keeping the limb attached to the prosthesis (its suspension). The initial evaluation and patient assessment then must be adequately in-depth to learn about all current safety concerns and also consider ahead of time all potential safety risks with the utilization of a new prosthetic or orthotic device – or rather, the utilization of all the components and design aspects of each device uniquely chosen for the older individual. Table 9.1 offers a summary of some of the prosthetic possibilities the practitioner begins with, before using clinical assessment data to identify a single-most ideal option; Table 9.2 highlights some potential questions the practitioner may consider during an appointment to develop the best prosthetic treatment plan.

When the evaluation takes place in the home setting, it becomes the additional responsibility of the clinician to observe the living environment and ask questions to confirm that all aspects of the patient's routine have been considered. Potential hazards such as steps, rug edges, and cords are visible in a shared walk-through of one's day, and the prosthetist-orthotist has the unique ability to highlight certain things such as the slipping hazard of an unshod ankle-foot orthosis or prosthetic foot on a tile floor [19, 20].

Such demonstrations would come up during a discussion of proper (and improper) uses of the device. It may not be intuitive to the average patient that most devices require the use of footwear at all times, even in the home. Aside from the risk of slipping, a change in alignment may occur when transitioning from shod to unshod conditions. A significant number of shoe options – for males and females alike – situate the heel in an elevated position compared to the sole of the foot, and prosthetic feet by default are typically built to assume a 3/8″ heel height in the shoe. When a patient removes a shoe from a device "aligned" to footwear with a specified heel height, there is the experience of closed chain biomechanical impacts, which can include knee hyperextension or the necessity to lean forward (flex) at the hip. There is evidence that minimal heel height is beneficial for the older patient, especially those at risk of falls [21], and a commitment to fully flat shoes potentially supports the continued use of a device even without shoes. Granted, making this possible with a lower limb orthosis takes strategic design with this end goal in mind-since many orthoses utilize the shoe as a critical part of its structure and function.

A crucial part of providing a prosthetic or orthotic device to a patient is alerting them to any and all safety considerations. This is an important step of the fitting and delivery process for any device, and the documentation of this patient education is rightfully expected by insurance payors as a prerequisite for payment and is a routine risk management step for the clinician and company alike. Aside from identifying proper and improper uses of the device, patients must also be oriented to the

Table 9.1 Design options for lower limb prosthetic intervention (not inclusive)

Socket design	Transtibial total surface bearing (TSB)
	Transtibial patellar tendon bearing (PTB)
	Transtibial hybrid design
	Transfemoral ischial containment
	Transfemoral sub-ischial
	Transfemoral quadrilateral
Method of interface	Sock ply
	Liner (TPE, silicone, urethane, etc.)
	Sheath
	Skin fit
Method of suspension	Belts/straps/joints
	Anatomical
	Locking
	Suction
Alignment considerations	Endoskeletal
	Exoskeletal
Knee unit (if applicable)	Fluid vs. non-fluid
	Microprocessor vs. non-microprocessor
	Single axis vs. polycentric
Foot/ankle system	Solid ankle cushion heel (SACH)
	Single axis
	Multiaxial
	Flexible keel
	Dynamic response
	Activity-specific
Education materials	Wear time (dosing) and device care guidelines
	Donning and doffing instructions
	Skin inspection
	Alignment considerations (shoe differences)
	Volume management

suggested methods of maintaining a device and its components and keeping them in working order, as well as the injuries that could take place with the use of the device. With these wear/care guidelines, patients are empowered to establish their own routine of inspection to look for anything on the device that could create problems or lead to component failure, as well as anything on their own body that is an early manifestation of device problems. Potential skin breakdown and the cascade of negative effects that follows are risks that are discussed with the provision of any product contacting a body segment, and the expectations of what a device failure could look like are always mentioned but are unique to each material and structural design. Special attention should be spent with the patient describing early observation of skin issues in the context of the patient's unique skin pigmentation.

Table 9.2 Questions assisting design selection for lower limb prosthetic intervention (general and not inclusive)

Socket	Was the procedure a transosseous or disarticulation amputation?
	Is the patient a previous prosthesis wearer?
	With what other comorbidities does this patient present?
	What medications is this patient using and potential side effects?
Interface	Are there any skin conditions or sensitivities present?
	How is the patient's upper extremity strength and dexterity?
	What is the level of cognition for this patient?
	Does the patient live alone or is there assisted care/family support?
Suspension	To what types of activities or occupation is the patient exposed?
	To what type of environment and climate is the patient exposed?
Alignment	To what type of occupation or activities is the patient exposed?
Knee	With what functional and cognitive abilities does the patient present?
	How long of a residual limb does this patient have?
Foot/ankle	To what type of activities, environment, and/or occupation is the patient exposed?
	What are the patient's health and life goals?
	How much clearance does this patient have?
	Are there any side effects from medications this patient might be on?
Componentry	To what other specific activities, exercises, or occupation will this patient be exposed?
	To what types of environments might this patient be exposed (i.e., harsh, corrosive, dry, humid, rainy)?

Thorough patient education includes the fact that injury as a result of device wear can occur acutely or manifest chronically and can happen at sites external to the body segments encompassed by any prosthetic or orthotic device. In the case of prostheses, interprofessional efforts of therapy throughout prosthetic rehabilitation are in part to address the attention and effort often required to help the older patient return to symmetry in gait; without this, the patient experiences increased risk of overuse or overstress injuries to the noninvolved side [22–24]. In the case of orthoses, a restriction in the range of motion at one or more joints often results in instances of hypermobility at one or more adjacent joints as the individual subconsciously explores compensatory movements to achieve similar outcomes in their routine activities. Contralateral overuse injury is a potential orthotic problem as well.

Evidence of prosthetic or orthotic problems does not always mean error on the user's part or the clinician's part. The human body changes over time, and the older human body is certainly no exception. Changes in physical condition are an eventual expectation. Changes in body weight and subsequent changes in limb volume can compromise the fit and function of a prosthesis or orthosis, and a change in activity level can have similar implications on function. The patient should understand what it means for a device to no longer fit, just like a caregiver should understand how a patient's decline in physical activity potentially changes the device requirements.

Crises are best averted at the earliest possible stages, and the prosthetist-orthotist requests involvement with any evidence or at any instinct of problem. Prosthetic and orthotic devices are rarely found to be intuitive for the older patient to manage independently, so it is important to provide adequate attention and clinical bandwidth to this population of patients – especially considering the fact that among a caseload of patients, these individuals are perhaps least proficient in the myriad means of communication mastered by younger generations. And just as the prosthetist-orthotist is acutely aware of the limitations in his or her scope of practice, it is also important that the patient recognizes the referring physician and other interprofessional partners as crucial resources when navigating emergencies and further health problems.

Finally, it should not be ignored that the home environment itself presents an entirely new set of hazards for the working clinical professional. Each home visited is different and may present unique challenges potentially hindering one's ability to provide adequate care. Safe and effective care is impacted by the ability to maintain standards for temperature, lighting, and sanitation; other authors have referenced negative environmental factors to include crowded or dimly lit surroundings, as well as socio-environmental factors such as family over- or under-involvement or limited access to supporting healthcare professionals [19].

Interprofessional Collaboration and Referrals/Coordinating Medical Services/Patient Selection of Services

Prosthetist-orthotists are members of the allied healthcare team, heavily reliant on the services of physicians and other specialists to initiate services and also to support parallel aspects of the patient's treatment plan. As a business, a clinic generates revenue by submitting insurance claims at the conclusion of patients' single episodes of care. Unlike most other entities doing business with health insurance companies in this way, prosthetic and orthotic organizations can only seek financial reimbursement for their services once care has concluded. Typically, this occurs when a finished device is officially provided to the patient to keep and is officially defined by paperwork notating a "delivery." As a result of this process, practitioners and their companies are investing time and energy and money up front, maintaining faith that they will be able to see the process through to its conclusion – so that a claim may ultimately be submitted on behalf of the patient/beneficiary. When home care is not an option, the treatment timeline can in some circumstances be stretched significantly, turning a weeks-long process into a months-long ordeal.

Prosthetic and orthotic clinicians can only provide services to individuals who have a physician's prescription defining their needs, and insurance paperwork typically requires them to get a secondary approval from the physician once a more specific plan can be nailed down in insurance-code language. Nonetheless, other healthcare professionals who work closely with physicians can be initiators of this process. As a result, these referral sources are not simply gatekeepers to potential customers but are partners in the treatment development process. Smart prosthetic and orthotic practitioners engage frequently with physicians and therapists in the design phase to ensure agreement as well as in follow-up to share positive outcomes. Maintaining a professional connection is important; there are countless reasons, for example, that referral back to their physician might be in order: for medication needs, to address wounds or pain, concern for mental health, etc.

Though the prosthetist-orthotist is usually recognized for his or her role in providing the patient with a new or updated device, the role of the professional is far more dynamic than being simply a supplier of medical equipment. Aside from all the customization of devices for optimal fit and the tuning or aligning of devices and their components for biomechanical efficiency, the clinician assesses for safety, educates on proper use and care, and trains individuals on how to make the best use of their new device as a tool. Frustratingly, the insurance-code language that defines clinical services and insurance coverage policies themselves only allows these clinicians and their organizations to be paid per device, per physical part, or for the time and labor involved in repairs thereof. This is in contrast to the use of Current Procedural Terminology (CPT) codes, which is afforded to most other healthcare providers; these codes reimburse professionals per service provided.

It therefore becomes crucial that the prosthetist-orthotist has a referring relationship with physical and occupational therapists and any other professionals that could support the multifaceted needs of the patient, especially when the patient is unknowing of those needs. An individual with new amputation will require therapy services in preparation for a prosthesis, as well as in prosthetic training after the fitting and delivery of the first prosthesis. But they may also require services at other times, when flexibility or strengthening needs become a limiting factor in the success of the patient's use of their device. In many cases, a properly designed prosthesis or orthosis does not immediately solve a clinical rehabilitation problem, and it becomes a professionally shared role to facilitate a patient's proper use of this new "tool" as they continue in the rehab process.

As with the selection of any service, the patient has the freedom to select their own provider for prosthetic and orthotic services. When making this choice, the older and home-restricted patient should feel empowered to ask many questions about what their treatment – and specifically their home-based treatment – will look like. It is fair and reasonable to inquire about what a device might look or feel like, about the timing of services, about expected financial responsibility, etc. When selecting among traditional clinical settings, patients typically work with the facility that is closest to their home. They may be ignorant in thinking that they are forced to utilize the services of the clinic either closest in proximity to their hospital or whose name and contact information was provided to them directly by the physician's office. Alternatively, when seeking home care services, the ability to be more selective among options may be more obvious. That said, mobile clinics and home care business models are the rarity, and an individual's list of in-network providers will ultimately be one of the main deciding factors if there are indeed multiple options. Anecdote would suggest that the patient care experience throughout the COVID-19 pandemic brought to light the need for more mobile clinic options, particularly in lesser-resourced and more rural regions. Many hope that this option will expand, considering the fact that home rehabilitation has the potential to enhance the patient's autonomy, independence, and community reintegration [25].

Like other medical offices, prosthetic and orthotic clinics typically operate with one or more front-office professionals who work to coordinate patients' care – managing appointments and insurance communication, among other crucially important things. In the case of home care, the older individual can be rest assured that services are coordinated just the same through these very same individuals.

Tele-Health

The COVID-19 pandemic highlighted tele-health as a partial solution for when in-person appointments are prevented from occurring. Partial, in that these virtual appointments were certainly able to provide patients an opportunity to speak to their clinician – but with so much of the prosthetist-orthotist's work connected to a prosthesis or orthosis, not being able to have hands on the device for adjustment or modification becomes a limiting factor for progress. Recall that financial reimbursement for services only takes place with the physical "delivery" of a device or with hands-on repair services, so tele-health appointments as a service are by definition not individually billable.

Now with the pandemic mostly behind us, clinics have recognized that tele-health can be applied strategically to benefit the patient and practitioner. The pattern of follow-up appointments in prosthetics and orthotics is not standardized and often varies by device and based on other characteristics or factors about the patient. Follow-up in general is very much a standard practice to ensure the longterm success of treatment, so clinics may use phone or virtual calls as an initial screening for what the patient will need in an upcoming in-person visit or to determine if the patient will need to come in at all. Recall again that the clinic likely receives no payment for a visit in which no services are needed – and a patient would certainly question the purpose of their visit if, in hindsight, nothing at all was necessary.

Tele-health may offer itself similarly as a tool for the mobile practitioner, seeking confirmation and clarification of needs from patients before arranging the logistics of an at-home visit. This may occur as simply as a phone call, but video capabilities could offer much more for the clinician's understanding. And yet, for the older patient, the many technological options to accomplish this feat may be out of reach. Perhaps the patient does not have a computer with a camera or does not know how to manage certain virtual communication applications. As with nearly everything at the practitioner's disposal in the field of prosthetics and orthotics, tele-health is yet another tool to utilize specifically when and where it can offer benefits.

Case Study: Perspective of a Prosthetist

The case study from Chap. 3 introduces us to Jeralean, a 75-year-old African American woman presenting with right lower limb amputation distal to the knee. Her need for amputation clearly arose from the effects of dysvascular disease, and it is apparent that the threat of amputation has not gone away. She maintains a long list of comorbidities (hypertension, diabetes, glaucoma, sleep apnea, constipation, neuropathy, osteoarthritis, and bouts of pneumonia) and an even longer list of medications (as many as 11 administered in a day). Her changes in appetite, weight, and mental health, combined with poor compliance with medications and prosthetic care, are potentially troubling. The logistical challenges of traveling over 60 miles to receive healthcare services suggest an obvious need for and potential benefit from home care services.

Diabetes increases one's amputation risk by 15–20 times, and with a higher proportional prevalence of diabetes, minority population groups such as African Americans are more likely to require amputation compared to other groups. It has been reported that half of individuals with diabetes-related amputations will undergo contralateral limb amputation 2–5 years following the initial procedure [26, 37]. Jeralean's risk is elevated due to her frailty. Electing to not wear her prosthesis, her upright mobility relies upon hopping around and navigating with the handheld support of structures and furniture around her – even the use of a walker would require utilization of her painful and stiff wrists and fingers. Her falls can certainly be attributed to this, with her body weight supported by only one distal limb. When a lower limb prosthesis is not used in standing and ambulation, forces and pressures through the contralateral foot double by default, made worse when neuropathy compromises protective sensation and joint proprioception, when pain symptoms arise from chronic arthritis, and certainly when progression of the diabetes disease compromises the sense of vision. One's base of support is severely limited with only one distal extremity contacting the ground, which gives even the smallest of transfers (sit to stand, bed to chair, etc.) enhanced fall risk. Cuts on her limbs introduce the possibility of infection, which may progress unknowingly due to peripheral neuropathy. Unless major changes are realized for Jeralean, she will undoubtedly require additional amputation as a means to save her life.

This patient requires a treatment plan with a goal of limiting excessive pressures and forces on the intact limb. She needs a mobility solution involving either an assistive device (wheelchair or walker) or a new prosthesis, likely both. The prosthetist would spend significant time with Jeralean exploring why she has chosen to no longer wear her prosthesis. A reasonable leading assumption would be that her weight loss over the last 6 months has resulted in proportional volume loss in her residual limb, compromising fit in the prosthetic socket. Perhaps as well her regimen of medications impacts fluid retention in her limbs or else carries side effects that make her feel unsafe while upright (without assistive devices). Perhaps the progression of vision loss or impaired upper limb dexterity has dramatically limited her ability to manage routine care and use of her prosthesis. The prosthetist responsible for providing her original device would have the ability to compare current subjective and objective observations with baseline data from the original evaluation.

Though prosthetists recognize the prosthetic device and treatment as their most primary care responsibility, the success of this intervention is very much reactive to common home care challenges related to the patient. One study organized these into categories of affective challenges, cognitive lack of knowledge, cognitive impairment/memory limitation, and physical challenges [20]. Jeralean's current mental health status results in her pushing away professional and interpersonal support, and so addressing this issue is paramount for prosthetic intervention to follow. Jeralean may feel this way due to a lack of knowledge regarding the many complex health situations she has been enduring, complicated by the recent passing of her spouse. As an interprofessional team, her healthcare providers should recommend counseling services and may seek an empathic approach to cut through any stigma that this carries within her generational and ethno-racial culture. Physician and pharmacist coordination should inform other professionals of her cognitive state and medication needs, and physical and occupational therapist coordination should inform colleagues of current and potential functional capabilities. All of this must be taken into consideration before deciding if prosthetic care continues to be appropriate.

Pharmacy Services

An important component of the clinical evaluation for the prosthetist-orthotist is the patient's self-report of medications taken, plus any additional information to be gained from physician notes regarding pharmacological intervention. Utilization of prescription drugs is common for the geriatric prosthetic or orthotic patient, considering the presentation of their underlying conditions. For prosthetic patients, pain management is a primary concern, and this potential pain can be categorized into residual limb pain versus phantom limb sensation and pain. The former often requires the careful use of opioid and narcotic analgesics – with attention to addiction prevention – while the latter demonstrates poor response to these more traditional pain management tactics. Often, the patient with amputation will require the involvement of anti-seizure or antidepressant medication to dampen or eliminate these more abstract versions of pain. While residual limb pain is more mechanical in nature – the body's natural response to damaged tissue, increased pressures, etc. – phantom sensation and pain arise from errant electrical signaling now that peripheral nerves have been severed from their original destinations. The brain's attempt to make sense of this input results in unusual sensations appearing to come from now-missing anatomy and ranging from bothersome to variations and episodes of excruciating pain [26].

Effective pain management is an obvious need for any patient, let alone the older homebound patient, due to the significant physiological stress and disruptions to homeostasis experienced by the body as a result of pain. All members of the healthcare team are certainly impacted by its negative impact on the patient's ability to concentrate and learn, and the prosthetist-orthotist would be quick to point out the impact of pain on mobility and rehabilitation progress. If the geriatric patient has just undergone amputation surgery, he or she must learn how to live in their "new normal" with a cautious monitoring eye looking out for infection and skin breakdown and additional attention yet to proper limb positioning and the controlling of any swelling. Pain can easily disrupt the patient in these responsibilities. With the potential to be fatiguing and demoralizing, it may come as no surprise that the success of early rehabilitation is positively influenced by effective postoperative pain management [20].

For the orthotic patient, there is a wide range of potential pharmacological needs, diagnosis- and presentation-specific. Reduction of spastic hypertonicity is an important component of the multidisciplinary treatment plan for the management of neuromuscular impairments, which alone can be addressed via numerous different drugs administered by oral, injection, or intrathecal means. Each method has a different timeline of effectiveness as well as its own list of potential adverse effects. Prescribed drug use in prosthetics and orthotics typically risks one or many of the following: drowsiness, dizziness, fatigue, weakness, nausea, and/or headache – plus countless others. Those highlighted here represent effects that can compromise the safe use of a device.

For medication intervention in general, the physician and pharmacist play very important roles on the interprofessional healthcare team, and this can only be more emphasized for the older patient in the home care setting. Among modernized nations, it has been observed that over half of seniors in home care use over five medications, with nearly a quarter using over eight [27]. In addition, the 13% of the US population 65 and over has been assessed to consume around 32% of all prescription drugs [28]. Pharmacists who prescribe for the geriatric population benefit from shared knowledge from all home care disciplines. This knowledge fosters an understanding of the unique needs of a complex population of individuals who consume multiple medications and manage multiple health conditions. Pharmacists apply this knowledge for the purpose of drug efficacy and safety [25, 29].

Despite patients and members of the healthcare team routinely demonstrating satisfaction with clinical pharmacy services [30], some have observed a high prevalence of inappropriate drug-taking behavior and pharmaceutical mismanagement [31, 32]. While pharmacy home visits are a readily available service to the older patient, pharmacists have not traditionally been recognized as members of home care teams [26]. Medication evaluations can be completed either by a pharmacist or prescribing physician. Evaluations conducted in combination with a comprehensive evaluation aids proper selection of type and dosage [29]. In fact, in-home pharmacy assessments offer the best opportunity to discover any problems with drug administration and use, given the array of complex medication regimens used in this population [27, 29].

During visits to the home, the pharmacist is able to observe patients' daily medication routine as well as the system they are employing to organize their medications. As with prosthetics and orthotics, each visit is an opportunity to reeducate patients on the purposes and administration of drugs, which can increase patients' understanding and compliance. Clinical eyes on the patient's drug supply allows the professional to recommend removal or discontinuation of expired or unnecessary medications – or ones that negatively interact – which can simplify their medication regimen. Pharmacists are adept at discussing with patients expected outcomes from the use of multiple prescription drugs, what side effects are reasonable to expect, how over-the-counter medications interact with prescribed medications, and when to reach out to the pharmacist [29].

Durable Medical Equipment

Patients utilizing home health services are more likely to utilize durable medical equipment (DME) services compared to prosthetic and orthotic services, though in many cases their needs include both. The Centers for Medicare & Medicaid Services (CMS) collectively categorize durable medical equipment and prosthetic and orthotic services as DMEPOS, but they are notably different in how they are provided to the patient. Considering the fact that DME can be found entirely prefabricated or one-size-fits-all, these services are often provided in a retail-type environment – though transactions can include rental payments or complete purchases. Broadly, DME is equipment that helps the patient to complete activities of daily living. It can include mobility-assisting devices (canes, walkers, wheelchairs) as well as many other types of items for use in the home (hospital beds, commodes, electrical stimulation units, portable oxygen equipment, etc.) [33, 34] . Like prosthetic and orthotic services, DME requires a prescription from a physician, and there are insurance-specific requirements and limitations to what receives coverage and when.

Regarding mobility concerns, assistive devices are observed to be effective at offsetting some of the effects of chronic disability. Despite this, it has been measured that less than half of chronically disabled individuals receive any DME at all through Medicare, suggesting dramatic underuse of an important resource for rehabilitative success [35]. Other studies have concluded that the most prominent barriers to obtaining mobility devices are challenges in navigating the process, inadequate insurance coverage, and lack of knowledge of insurance benefits [36]. Considering this, home health medical professionals should recognize the shared responsibility of assessing a patient's needs for mobility equipment or other DME that could improve the rehabilitative process as well as improve their quality of life.

Those that do receive DME in the home may be benefitting from recent decades of technology innovation, perhaps utilizing things like infusion pumps, dialysis machines, blood glucose meters, powered wheelchairs, etc. While this expansion of access is greatly beneficial, the original design of this equipment to be used in clinical settings by trained professionals means that their complexity may still present a barrier to the patient – and the healthcare professional may need an eye toward whether or not a piece of equipment is safe and functioning properly for the patient or if they may provide additional training and education for proper use [20, 29].

Nutritional Services

Maintaining optimal nutrition throughout the lifespan is essential for overall health and well-being. This becomes even more of a necessity as individuals age. The population of older adults faces unique challenges when it comes to meeting their nutritional needs, making it crucial to address specific considerations to promote healthy aging, vitality, and longevity as individuals approach the end stages of life. Physiological changes, decreased appetite, chronic health conditions, medication interactions, and social factors should all be considered when determining and managing the nutritional needs of older adults. When support teams can recognize these challenges, they will be better equipped to develop individualized nutrition care plans to support the nutritional needs of older adults. Remember – the goal of an individualized nutrition care plan is to not only meet the patient's physiological needs but to also encourage a positive relationship with food that in return fosters their vitality, independence, and quality of life.

The following are dietary considerations that may require referral to a registered dietitian:

- *Dental and Oral Health Issues*: Several studies show that older adults with impaired dentition and chewing ability (tooth loss, ill-fitting dentures, etc.) consume fewer calories. This can lead to inadequate caloric consumption for weight maintenance and physiological needs. Other studies show that dentures may alter the taste of food – which can impact food decisions in regard to food choice, intake, and nutritional quality.
- *Food Intake*: Inadequate food intake is the leading cause of malnutrition. Food increase usually decreases as age increases. You will see a decrease in macronutrients (carbohydrates, protein, and fats), but also, possibly more important to be aware of is the loss of consumption of micronutrients. In order to ensure a sufficient intake of essential vitamins and minerals, incorporating a multivitamin might be a feasible solution to compensate for the lack of nutrient-dense real food consumption.
- *Substance Abuse*: Alcohol abuse is a common, yet under-recognized, problem in older adults. Frequent, chronic alcohol use is associated with lower-quality nutrition due to a replacement of food for substance use. Chronic use or abuse can result in vitamin deficiencies.
- *Depression and Social Isolation*: Studies have shown that depression and loneliness can be a major factor in weight loss in nursing facilities or for those without social support. It is important to emphasize the importance of eating as a group, as it has been shown that social environments increase overall intake.

- *Hunger and Food Insecurity*: There is a relationship that exists between poverty, the older adult, and food adequacy. When working with older patients, consider the following three things – money, transportation, and preparation. As a practitioner, it is one thing to suggest a certain intake of foods, but if the patient does not have the money to afford it, the transportation to access it, and a means to prepare it safely, then the suggestions mean nothing. Become aware of food assistance programs such as the Supplemental Nutrition Assistance Program, home-delivered meals, food pantries, and Commodity Supplemental Food Program.

Many medical diagnoses also require nutritional considerations. Examples include Alzheimer's, CVD, CKD, COPD, constipation, diabetes, osteoporosis, and pressure ulcers. Management of these conditions should be overseen by a registered dietitian. Additionally, a micronutrient deficiency may be detected by physically observing the older adult. Deficiencies frequently present in the hair, eyes, lips, gums, teeth, tongue, face, neck, skin, gastrointestinal tract, muscular system, skeletal system, and nervous system [38].

Case Study: Perspective of a Registered Dietician

It is noteworthy to mention that when a client is nearing the end of life, it is important that nutrition goals match the medical goals of the patient (restorative, supportive, palliative, or comfort). Patients have the right to refuse nutrition and hydration. In regard to the case study "Jeralean," the registered dietician nutritionist would take the following actions:

- Discuss with Jeralean her eating habits and rate of weight loss – 20 pounds within 6 months.
- Ascertain more information pertaining to food insecurity, food procurement, food accessibility, and food preparation ability.
- Discuss sleep hygiene (e.g., latest caffeine intake, big meals or meal sizes, bedroom temperature and lighting).
- Conduct a medicine evaluation to see if weight loss is attributed to high blood sugars.
- Perform a nutrition focused physical exam to possibly identify any micronutrient/macronutrient deficiencies (in conjunction with the physician).
- Review available healthcare records.
- Share findings and consult with other care team members, as needed.
- Remain available for consultations with other care team members.

Chapter Summary

Prosthetic and orthotic services are valuable for patients with amputations and those requiring support for musculoskeletal impairments. Pharmacy services are beneficial for patients needing assistance with medication organization, medication monitoring, medication administration, and medication adherence. Durable medical equipment services are useful for older adults who require physical medical equipment within the home setting to assist with a better quality of living. Lastly, nutritional services are frequently needed to assure that the nutritional needs of the patient are being addressed.

Discussion Question

1. Consider the following: Your patient demonstrates the ability to don and doff the device properly; however, when therapy arrives, you notice the patient constantly has their prosthesis removed. What are some recommendations that could be provided to the patient to ensure compliance?

Multiple Choice Questions

1. Which of the following dietary conditions may *not* require referral to a registered dietician?
   (a) Tonsillitis
   (b) Ill-fitting dentures
   (c) Chronic alcohol use
   (d) Depression
2. Micronutrient deficiencies can be physically observed in which of the body's structures?
   (a) Hair
   (b) Muscular system
   (c) Skeletal system
   (d) All of the above
3. Examples of durable medical equipment include all but which of the following?
   (a) Blood glucose meters
   (b) Wheelchairs
   (c) Dialysis machine
   (d) Shower chair

4. Which of the following is a primary concern for prosthetic patients?
   (a) Sweat management
   (b) Sock management
   (c) Pain management
   (d) Range of motion

5. Which of the following may present a challenge for the orthotist in the home setting?
   (a) Overprotective family members
   (b) Working with minimal tools
   (c) The presence of small children in the home
   (d) Poor air quality in the home

6. What care model do prosthetists and orthotists adhere to?
   (a) National Care Model (NCM)
   (b) Prosthetic and Orthotic Quality Care Framework (POQCF)
   (c) International Classification of Functioning, Disability and Health (ICF)
   (d) None of the above

Please refer to Table 9.1 and Table 9.2 to complete this assignment. The assignment applies to the case study in Chap. 2.

Consider Jeralean, and summarize the findings and potential considerations that the healthcare team must consider when working with this patient. Think back to the home environment and potential obstacles that the patient might encounter. What other factors or considerations would you advise the patient on, for example, referral for other health conditions or considerations?

References

1. American Board for Certification in Orthotics, Prosthetics & Pedorthics, Inc. (2022, September). *Practice analysis of certified practitioners in the disciplines of orthotics and prosthetics.* https://www.abcop.org/docs/default-source/practice-analyses/abc-practitioner-practiceanalysis-2022.pdf?sfvrsn=7a79667d_13
2. Prince, M. J., Wu, F., Guo, Y., Robledo, L. M. G., O'Donnell, M., Sullivan, R., & Yusuf, S. (2015). The burden of disease in older people and implications for health policy and practice. *The Lancet, 385*(9967), 549–562.
3. Kahle, J. T., & Highsmith, J. M. (2008). Barriers limiting the geriatric client from accessing orthotic care. *Topics in Geriatric Rehabilitation, 24*(4), 332–336.
4. Highsmith, M. J. (2008). Barriers to the provision of prosthetic Services in the Geriatric Population. *Topics in Geriatric Rehabilitation, 24*(4), 325–331.
5. McDougall, J., Wright, V., & Rosenbaum, P. (2010). The ICF model of functioning and disability: Incorporating quality of life and human development. *Developmental Neurorehabilitation, 13*(3), 204–211.
6. Russell, D., Mola, A., Onorato, N., Johnson, S., Williams, J., Andaya, M., & Flannery, M. (2017). Preparing home health aides to serve as health coaches for home care patients with chronic illness: Findings and lessons learned from a mixed-method evaluation of two pilot programs. *Home Health Care Management & Practice, 29*(3), 191–198.

7. Shamus, E., Fabrizi, S., & Hogan, J. (2018). A qualitative study of professional issues in home health therapy. *Home Health Care Management & Practice, 30*(1), 9–15.
8. Webster, J. B., & Murphy, D. P. (2019). *Atlas of orthoses and assistive devices*. Elsevier Health Sciences.
9. Dickinson, A. S., Donovan-Hall, M. K., Kheng, S., Bou, K., Tech, A., Steer, J. W., et al. (2022). Selecting appropriate 3D scanning technologies for prosthetic socket design and transtibial residual limb shape characterization. *JPO: Journal of Prosthetics and Orthotics, 34*(1), 33–43.
10. Ramsdell, J. W. (1991). Geriatric assessment in the home. *Clinics in Geriatric Medicine, 7*(4), 677–694.
11. Heinemann, A. W., Connelly, L., Ehrlich-Jones, L., & Fatone, S. (2014). Outcome instruments for prosthetics: Clinical applications. *Physical Medicine and Rehabilitation Clinics, 25*(1), 179–198.
12. Shirley Ryan Ability Lab. (2023). *Rehabilitation measures database*. https://www.sralab.org/rehabilitation-measures.
13. de Niet MSc, M., van Duijnhoven, H. J., & Geurts, A. C. (2008). Falls in individuals with stroke. *Journal of Rehabilitation Research and Development, 45*(8), 1195.
14. Watanabe, Y. (2005). Fear of falling among stroke survivors after discharge from inpatient rehabilitation. *International Journal of Rehabilitation Research, 28*(2), 149–152.
15. Mackintosh, S. F., Hill, K., Dodd, K. J., Goldie, P., & Culham, E. (2005). Falls and injury prevention should be part of every stroke rehabilitation plan. *Clinical Rehabilitation, 19*(4), 441–451.
16. Macgilchrist, C., Paul, L., Ellis, B. M., Howe, T. E., Kennon, B., & Godwin, J. (2010). Lower-limb risk factors for falls in people with diabetes mellitus). *Diabetic Medicine, 27*(2), 162–168.
17. DeMott, T. K., Richardson, J. K., Thies, S. B., & Ashton-Miller, J. A. (2007). Falls and gait characteristics among older persons with peripheral neuropathy. *American Journal of Physical Medicine & Rehabilitation, 86*(2), 125–132.
18. Dite, W., Connor, H. J., & Curtis, H. C. (2007). Clinical identification of multiple fall risk early after unilateral transtibial amputation. *Archives of Physical Medicine and Rehabilitation, 88*(1), 109–114.
19. Gershon, R. R., Dailey, M., Magda, L. A., Riley, H. E., Conolly, J., & Silver, A. (2012). Safety in the home healthcare sector: Development of a new household safety checklist. *Journal of Patient Safety, 8*(2), 51–59.
20. Beer, J. M., McBride, S. E., Mitzner, T. L., & Rogers, W. A. (2014). Understanding challenges in the front lines of home health care: A human-systems approach. *Applied Ergonomics, 45*(6), 1687–1699.
21. Menant, J. C., Steele, J. R., Menz, H. B., Munro, B. J., & Lord, S. R. (2008). Optimizing footwear for older people at risk of falls.
22. Privratsky, A. B. (2008). Do prosthetists see a benefit in having "in-house" physical therapy Services for Patients with Amputation? *JPO: Journal of Prosthetics and Orthotics, 20*(2), 61–66.
23. Shih, H. T., Kubo, M. M., Horn, L. D., Gorton, J. N., Ferraro, A. L., MacLeod, T. D., & Lee, S. P. (2022). Patient experience and perceived benefits of physical therapy after lower limb amputation in middle-aged and older adults. *Journal of Allied Health, 51*(3), 180–191.
24. Devinuwara, K., Dworak-Kula, A., & O'Connor, R. J. (2018). Rehabilitation and prosthetics postamputation. *Orthopaedics and Traumatology, 32*(4), 234–240.
25. Portnow, J., Kline, T., Daly, M. A., Peltier, S. M., Chin, C., & Miller, J. R. (1991). Multidisciplinary home rehabilitation. A practical model. *Clinics in Geriatric Medicine, 7*(4), 695–706.
26. Chui, K. C., Jorge, M., Yen, S. C., & Lusardi, M. M. (2020). *Orthotics and prosthetics in rehabilitation*. Saunders.
27. Fialová, D., & Desplenter, F. (2016). Aging of the population, clinical pharmacy services, and interdisciplinary cooperation in the optimization of pharmacotherapy in older patients. *Drugs & Aging, 33*(3), 163–167.

28. French, E. H. (1994). Adverse drug reactions and metabolic changes in the elderly. *US Pharmacist, 19*, H6–H16.
29. Mitzner, T. L., Beer, J. M., McBride, S. E., Rogers, W. A., & Fisk, A. D. (2009, October). Older adults' needs for home health care and the potential for human factors interventions. In *Proceedings of the human factors and ergonomics society annual meeting* (Vol. 53, No. 11, pp. 718–722). SAGE Publications.
30. MacAulay, S., Saulnier, L., & Gould, O. (2008). Provision of clinical pharmacy services in the home to patients recently discharged from hospital: A pilot project. *Canadian Journal of Hospital Pharmacy, 61*(2).
31. Willcox, S. M., Himmelstein, D. U., & Woolhandler, S. (1994). Inappropriate drug prescribing for the community-dwelling elderly. *JAMA, 272*(4), 292–296.
32. Der, E. H., Rubenstein, L. Z., & Choy, G. S. (1997). The benefits of in-home pharmacy evaluation for older persons. *Journal of the American Geriatrics Society, 45*(2), 211–214.
33. Wolff, J. L., Agree, E. M., & Kasper, J. D. (2005). Wheelchairs, walkers, and canes: What does Medicare pay for, and who benefits? *Health Affairs, 24*(4), 1140–1149.
34. Romanoski, N., & Swope, K. (2018). Durable medical equipment that supports activities of daily living, transfers and ambulation. In *The American Academy of physical medicine and rehabilitation*. PM&R Knowledge Now.
35. Iwashyna, T. J., & Christie, J. D. (2007). Low use of durable medical equipment by chronically disabled elderly. *Journal of Pain and Symptom Management, 33*(3), 324–330.
36. Cohen, L. J., & Perling, R. (2015). Barriers to mobility device access. *Topics in Geriatric Rehabilitation, 31*(1), 19–25.
37. Krajbich, J. I., Pinzur, M. S., Potter, B. K., & Stevens, P. M. (2023). *Atlas of amputations & limb deficiencies*. Wolters Kluwer Health.
38. Piland, C., Adams K., (Eds.) (2009). Pocket resource for nutrition assessment. In *Dietetics in health care communities* (pp. 65–69). American Dietetic Association.

Chapter 10
Conclusion: Integration and Synthesis

Danita H. Stapleton and Sekeria Bossie

Learning Objectives

1. Integrate theoretical frameworks and models that are fundamental to the delivery of effective home healthcare services.
2. Describe procedures for implementing and maintaining quality service delivery.
3. Explain interprofessional team members' contributions to home care delivery.
4. Identify critical aspects of interprofessional teaming and collaborations.

Introduction

Interprofessional team collaboration is central to providing effective and quality care within the home setting for older adults. This book provided a medium for learning more about the various roles and functions of interprofessional team members and their best care practices. Legislation, policy, and theoretical care perspectives were presented, as well as content pertaining to professional ethics, multicultural issues, quality of life issues, health literacy, assessment, safety considerations, and crisis planning. Other essential aspects of collaborative care practices were also discoursed. Central to any interprofessional team is the patient. The family also has a pivotal function in the care process. All care interventions must be planned,

Supplementary Information The online version contains supplementary material available at https://doi.org/10.1007/978-3-031-40889-2_10.

D. H. Stapleton (✉) · S. Bossie
Department of Rehabilitation Studies, College of Health Sciences, Alabama State University, Montgomery, AL, USA
e-mail: dstapleton@alasu.edu; sbossie@alasu.edu

D. H. Stapleton, S. Bossie (eds.), *Home Care for Older Adults Using Interprofessional Teams*, https://doi.org/10.1007/978-3-031-40889-2_10

implemented, and monitored (by interprofessional team members) with the best interest of the patient (and family, as appropriate) in mind.

Integration and Synthesis of Diverse Care Perspectives

Figure 10.1 depicts collective care aspects from the varied theoretical care models and frameworks presented in this book. It is noteworthy to mention that no single model or framework can adequately capture all facets of quality and effective home healthcare delivery. Thus, Fig. 10.1 portrays only a few essential features that were consistently highlighted in the previous chapters. These features have roots in biopsychosocial approaches, systems theory, ecological theory, ICG care framework, and the IPEC model of care. These features are dynamic and interactive, all impacting the patient and patient care outcomes. Patient care outcomes are influenced by a myriad of actions and decisions executed by IP team members. In Fig. 10.1, the skills and functions surrounding the patient (at center) are hallmarks of interprofessional collaboration. The authors of this chapter strongly assert that there is a positive correlation between patients' health outcomes and the active and continuous presence of the core competencies indicated in Fig. 10.1.

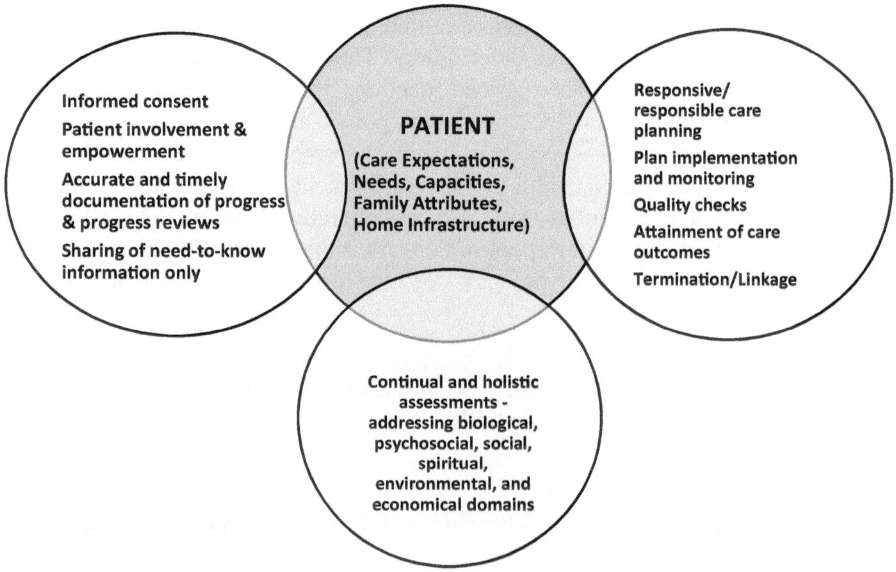

Fig. 10.1 A depiction of the integration and synthesis of multiple care competencies. These guide the provision of interprofessional home care for older patients

Maximizing Health Outcomes for Older Patients

Listed below are 11 provider-specific actions that clearly maximize interprofessional team collaboration. This is not an all-inclusive list. However, it is the hope of the authors that the list will continue to evolve for the betterment of patients, families, and interprofessional team members.

1. The IP team member must be willing to learn from other IP team members.
2. The IP team member must commit to making the following care aspects a priority: patient education (health literacy) and IP team member education (discipline literacy).
3. The IP team member must be willing to prioritize communication and to maintain cordial and cooperative relationships with the patient, family, and other IP team members.
4. The IP team member must be accessible and responsive to the needs of the entire IP team.
5. The IP team member must embrace the power of a holistic assessment and view it as a continuous care obligation.
6. The IP team member must be committed to familiarizing oneself with the ethical codes and obligations of other IP team members.
7. The IP team member must strive to be ethical in all aspects of care.
8. The IP team member must commit to resolving differences of opinions and perspectives expediently and in the best interest of the patient.
9. The IP team member must embrace principles of accountability and transparency, thus regularly engaging in quality improvement endeavors to assure quality patient care and patient satisfaction.
10. The IP team member must commit to fully implementing the care plan and engaging in timely and accurate reporting.
11. The IP team member must display humility at all times and not hesitate to ask for guidance or clarification when needed. This includes actively soliciting feedback about performance and the effectiveness of interventions.

Mindfully carrying out these required actions will maximize health outcomes for older patients receiving home healthcare services. These competencies are the basis for patient-centered care, quality treatment, and successful interprofessional collaborations.

Communication Is Fundamental

Two primary types of communication transpire between IP team members: synchronous and asynchronous. Synchronous communication refers to a collaboration in which members exchange information in real time (e.g., face-to-face, telephone, videoconferencing software such as Zoom or Microsoft Teams). Asynchronous communication refers to collaboration that does not occur in real time and occurs through the use of email messages or technological software such as a healthcare portal. In many cases, IP team members will use both synchronous and asynchronous methods of collaboration. For instance, the IP team might hold initial meetings synchronously but chose to communicate asynchronously for the duration of care. Regardless of the communication mode, IP team members must agree to communicate routinely, effectively, and transparently.

A Best Practice Quality Model for Home Care Services

The academic literature has defined quality of care as the "degree to which a set of inherent characteristics fulfills requirements" [1]. The Institute of Medicine (National Academy of Medicine) rendered the following definition – "…the degree to which health services for individuals and populations increase the likelihood of desired health outcomes and are consistent with current professional knowledge" – and further outlined the six domains of quality of care: safety, effectiveness, patient-centeredness, timeliness, efficiency, and equity [2, 3]. The authors of this book have adopted their own definition of quality of care:

> The term "quality of care" is best defined as an important practice concept that drives: (a) care planning; (b) patient engagement, progress, and satisfaction; and (c) the conscientious work of interprofessional team members. The term *conscientious* characterizes a team member who is: (a) reliable, punctual, accountable, and ethical; (b) discerning of patient needs and strengths and patient risk and protective factors; and (c) committed to adhering to agency policies and procedures. Quality of care is accomplished when the three aforementioned criteria are met by each member of the interprofessional team.

Table 10.1 and Fig. 10.2 portray aspects of a best practice (quality) model for home healthcare. This model has five phases that are intended to guide the conscientious IP team member in "checking for quality" throughout the episode of home care. This simple model warrants a "yes" or "no" response to several fundamental quality indicators. A "yes" response specifies that a quality indicator has been accomplished. Similarly, a "no" response specifies that a quality indicator is lacking or has not been accomplished. Any "no" responses should result in the team member executing at least two of the following decisive actions: (1) Enter a detailed progress note in the patient record explaining the identification of the issue and the plan for addressing the issue (a follow-up entry should address resolution); (2) discuss the issue with the IP team and referral source (document in the patient record the purpose of the meeting/consultation and the outcome); and (3) discuss the issue with the patient and family members (document the purpose of the discussion and the outcome). Quality checks are just as important in the healthcare industry as they are in other industries. These quality examinations are systematic and instrumental in maintaining desired levels of service quality at every stage of the care delivery process. They are determinants of whether services meet the requirements of the industry, agency, and patient and family.

Table 10.1 "Checking for quality" throughout the episode of care

Phase 1 – receipt of referral for care provision
Yes/no – contact made with patient/client via telephone within 2 business days
Yes/no – contact made with other IP team members within 5 business days
Yes/no/N/A – review code of ethics for IP team members within 10 business days (particularly if this is the first time working with a member or discipline)
Yes/no – research issues pertaining to patient/family cultural status within 5 business days of referral
Phase 2 – care planning/development
Yes/no – meeting convened with patient and other IP team members within 10 business days of referral
Yes/no – initial meeting had the following components: introduction of patient and family; introduction of professionals to include a description of their role, purpose, and anticipated benefits of their interventions
Yes/no – patient/family was assisted in articulating care needs
Yes/no – patient/family had opportunities to ask questions
Yes/no – patient/family was made aware of patient/client rights and grievance procedures
Yes/no – privacy and confidentiality parameters were explicitly addressed
Yes/no – patient/family was active in care planning and plan development
Yes/no – a unified plan was developed for patient assessment and treatment
Yes/no – informed consent was discussed and health literacy provided
Yes/no – care goals are functional and SMART
Yes/no – preservice assessment information is shared, if applicable
Yes/no – IP team members exchanged contact information and agreed upon communication methods and frequencies
Yes/no – IP team members received signed consent forms from patient for the sharing of care information
Yes/no – IP team members and the patient/family discussed scheduling of in-home services and frequency of services
Yes/no – current patient and home safety issues are discussed/addressed; crisis situations and conditions are discussed/addressed
Yes/no – relevant cultural issues were solicited for discussion
Phase 3 – care implementation
Yes/no – discipline-based assessments occur initially and continuously
Yes/no – service frequency and duration are in accordance with the care plan
Yes/no – patient/family is notified promptly when IP member cannot arrive to the home as scheduled
Yes/no – any patient/family needs or concerns (e.g., conditions presenting imminent harm; signs of abuse, neglect, or maltreatment; signs of health deterioration, patient dissatisfaction, etc.) are promptly shared with IP team members through the agreed upon channels and with the appropriate legal authority or protective services entity
Yes/no – monthly review of care goals with patient and family (barriers to care are discussed with the patient, family, and IP team)
Yes/no – patient is consistently available for services
Yes/no – informed consent is provided for new procedures or activities

(continued)

Table 10.1 (continued)

Yes/no – the home environment is continuously assessed for possible confidentiality and privacy breaches
Yes/no – successful delivery, follow-through, or follow-up on commitments made to patient/family
Yes/no – monthly updates and timely emergency notifications to referring physician or referral source
Yes/no – accurate and timely reports and documentation
Yes/no – frequent checks for patient understanding and satisfaction
Yes/no – patient services and interactions promote good and prevent or minimize harm
Yes/no/N/A – caregiver burden is discussed and addressed
Yes/no – the home environment is continuously assessed for safety concerns
Phase 4 – interprofessional collaboration
Yes/no – IP team meetings occur at least monthly or at least two members of the IP team are updated at least monthly. IP meetings take place in the client/patient home when possible
Yes/no – collaborative decision-making or approval is apparent
Yes/no/N/A – IP team disputes and differences are communicated and resolved within 10 business days
Yes/no – relevant knowledge is shared, and communication is maximized with (no obvious barriers to information flow among team members)
Yes/no – care coordination is seamless
Yes/no – there is evidence of advocacy on behalf of the patient/family, particularly as it relates to normalization, community access and integration, and least restrictive care environments
Yes/no/N/A – caregiver burden is discussed and addressed
Phase 5 – service termination/closure
Yes/no – the IP team met for a final meeting before officially terminating in-home interventions
Yes/no – the patient/family was given the opportunity to report outcomes in their own words
Yes/no – there was a review of care plan goals and outcomes (reflections on patient progress)
Yes/no – there was documented linkage to relevant community services, resources, and supports
Yes/no – there was a distinct handoff of care delivery or care responsibility
Yes/no – patient/family was instructed to call for future assistance, as needed (e.g., deterioration of health status or the need for additional services)
Yes/no – feedback was solicited from the patient and family on the impact of IP collaboration

IP Team Members' (Practice) Contributions

Interprofessional collaboration can be defined as a process that involves communication, decision-making, and interactions between individuals with expert knowledge in various professional disciplines [4]. The composition of the IP team depends on the practice setting, the needs of the patient or client, and the care goals established. A primary goal of the IP team is to apply multiple perspectives in the treatment of a patient to assure that physical and emotional needs are met [5]. However, members can use their expert knowledge to address numerous issues impacting a patient's healthcare. IP teaming reduces the occurrence of service duplication, care

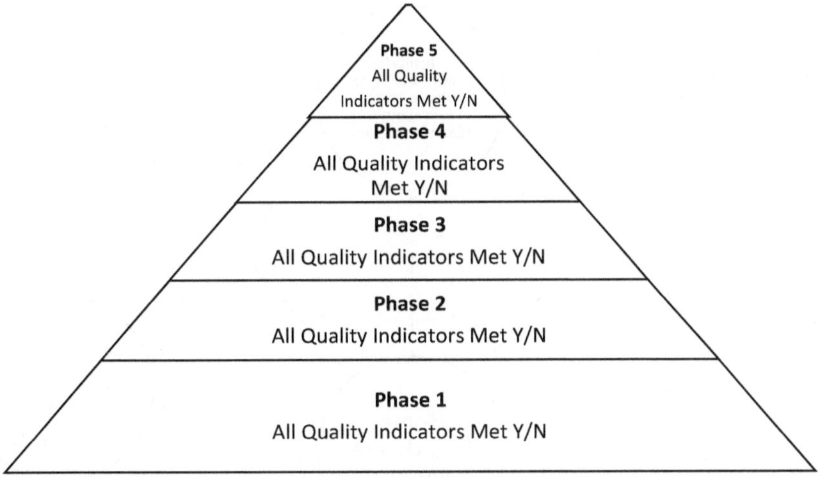

Fig. 10.2 Best practice "checking for quality" model. This pyramid represents the five phases of care. The phases align with the quality indicators depicted in Table 10.1. A "no" to any of the items will result in at least two decisive actions

fragmentation, and gaps in service delivery. IP members are major contributors to the continuum of care for older adults. A care continuum would not be possible without effective IP team dynamics and collaboration. Figure 10.3 synthesizes the functions of several IP team members who collaboratively contribute to the care continuum: physician, prosthetist and orthotist, pharmacist, nurse, social worker, physical therapist, occupational therapist, behavioral health professional, and registered dietician nutritionist. Many of these team members contributed to the formation of this book.

Interprofessional Team Collaboration Moving Forward: The Need for New Policy and Legislation

Proponents of interprofessional collaboration within the home care milieu must vocalize their positive (and not so positive) experiences at the local, state, and federal levels. They must advocate for government and corporate backing that will enable them to more flexibly meet the needs of older adults who desire to age at home and to do so with dignity. Timely and creative solutions are needed for older adults with limited family support and financial resources. Those residing in rural areas are in dire need of home healthcare services, particularly with the mass closing of hospitals in some rural areas. Consideration should be given to providing financial incentives to IP team members who desire to practice in rural areas. Additionally, there should be priority efforts focused on establishing quality standards and training for telehealth providers in order to minimize claims of

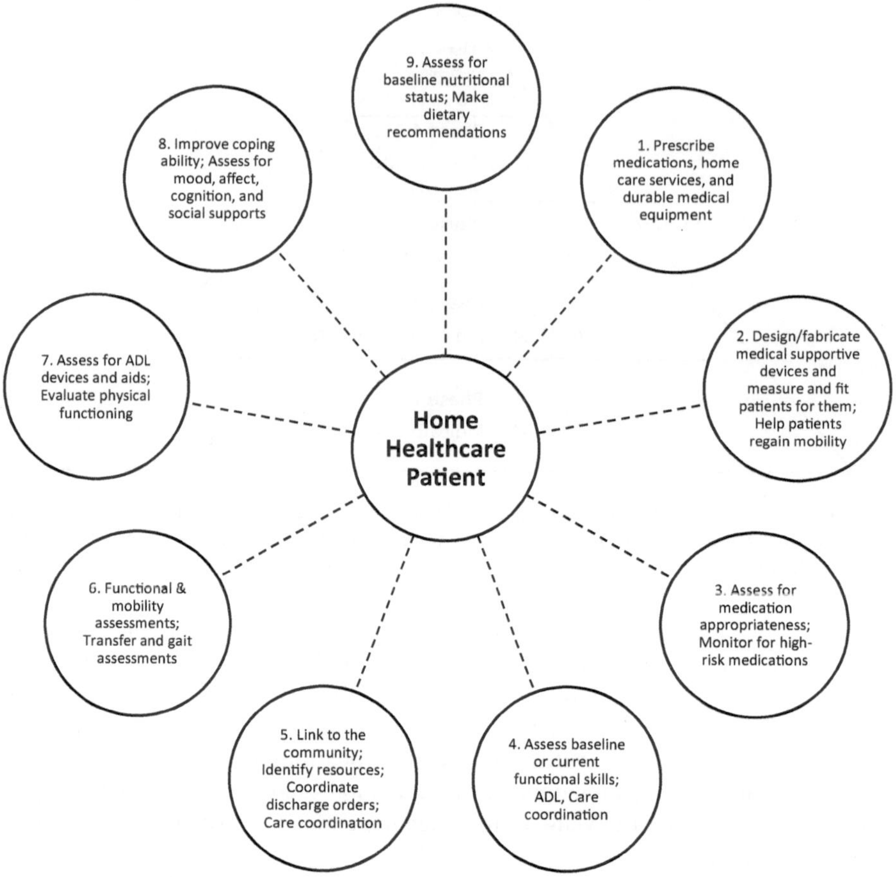

Fig. 10.3 Examples of interprofessional team members' home care contributions. Key: MD, 1; P&O, 2; PHA, 3; NRS, 4; SW, 5; PT, 6; OT, 7; BHP, 8; RDN, 9

negligence, exploitation, or malpractice. We conclude this chapter and the book with some final suggestions for action and policy change. It is our hope that these suggestions will serve as a basis for deeper discussions and dialogs between IP team members who champion the right of older adults to receive quality home care services.

- IP teams would benefit from technologies that allow for more direct and seamless communication amongst all providers who care for older patients in the home setting. Professionals from diverse agencies and disciplines would benefit from having one healthcare portal to enter timely reports and progress notes.
- More federal funds are needed to ensure the expansion of stable broadband connections in rural and underserved communities. Successful telehealth initiatives would reduce healthcare disparities for older individuals who are aging at

home in rural communities. These technologies would also make it possible for real-time virtual IP team meetings and consultations to be initiated successfully from the home setting.

- IP teams would benefit from policy changes related to Medicare coverage. Home care services are currently covered by Medicare for a limited period. In many instances, the time parameter does not permit for significant improvements to be noted in patients with complex medical needs. Extending Medicare coverage of home care from the typical 30 days to at least 90 days or longer would be advantageous for some patients. Additionally, Medicare needs to authorize more disciplines as "acceptable and skilled" providers of home healthcare.
- There should be mandates governing the frequency of contact between IP team members providing home care, particularly if the patient has complex medical needs. Collaborative endeavors such as consultations and interprofessional team meetings should be deemed billable services. Currently, many collaborations of this nature are not reimbursable. Allowing reimbursement for collaborative endeavors would send a strong message to the healthcare industry on the value of interprofessional collaboration.
- Lastly, more funding should be allocated for mobile units, particularly those providing behavioral health and prosthetic and orthotic services.

Chapter Summary

The overall theme of this book was to highlight the positive impact of interprofessional collaboration on the lives of older clients and patients in the home care setting. We wanted to use this book for *discipline literacy* and as a forum for understanding the inner workings of interprofessional collaboration. If applied and utilized effectively, interprofessional collaboration can foster a level of expertise about patients, families, and communities that will render dividends throughout the duration of a team member's career. The role of IP teams in the provision of services for older adults cannot be dismissed or devalued. Their roles will continue to evolve as the needs of patients, families, and communities evolve. More and more healthcare professionals are selecting home care as a practice option, and the results are stimulating. Our hope is that those reading this book will commit to collaborating respectfully with other disciplines and advocating strongly for older adults who desire home healthcare services.

Discussion Question

1. Compare and contrast the three definitions of "quality of care."

Multiple Choice Questions

1. All home care interventions must be planned, implemented, and monitored with the best interest of ___________ in mind.
   (a) The family
   (b) The patient
   (c) The interprofessional team
   (d) The patient and family
2. What is the primary objective of this book?
   (a) To increase the reader's knowledge of various healthcare disciplines
   (b) To increase the reader's knowledge of the health needs of older patients
   (c) To increase the reader's knowledge of the health needs of older patients from an interprofessional collaborative perspective
   (d) To increase the reader's knowledge of quality and best practices within the home care setting
3. Which of the following principles of care should continue throughout the episode of care, from the initial visit until care termination?
   (a) Informed consent
   (b) Quality assurance activities
   (c) Timely and accurate documentation and reporting
   (d) All of the above
4. Which of the following is an example of asynchronous communication?
   (a) Communication via a healthcare portal
   (b) Zoom meeting
   (c) Phone conference
   (d) In-person meeting
5. Ideally, a service quality check should be conducted
   (a) During each home visit
   (b) At least monthly
   (c) At least quarterly
   (d) During discharge

References

1. Hoyle, D. (2009). *ISO 9000 quality systems handbook: Using the standards as a framework for business improvement*. Elsevier.
2. IOM. (1990). In K. N. Lohr (Ed.), *Medicare: A strategy for quality assurance*. National Academic Press.

3. Institute of Medicine (IOM). (2001). *Crossing the quality Chasm. A new health system for the 21st century.* Volume 2001 National Academy Press.
4. Bridges, D. R., Davidson, R. A., Odegard, P. S., Maki, I. V., & Tomkowiak, J. (2011). Interprofessional collaboration: Three best practice models of interprofessional education. *Medical Education, 16.*
5. Peltonen, J., Leino-Kilpi, H., Heikkilä, H., Rautava, P., Tuomela, K., Siekkinen, M., et al. (2020). Instruments measuring interprofessional collaboration review. *Journal of Interprofessional Care, 34*(2), 147–161.

Appendices

Appendix A: Answer Key

Chapter 1

Discussion Question

1. Explain the significance of quality measures and measures of quality assurance in healthcare systems:

    Varied Response

D. H. Stapleton, S. Bossie (eds.), *Home Care for Older Adults Using Interprofessional Teams*, https://doi.org/10.1007/978-3-031-40889-2

Multiple Choice Questions

1. What legislation aided patients in leaving the hospital to recover at home with a mix of expanded services such as skilled nursing therapy, personal care, telehealth services, and more?
    (a) **Choose Home Care Act** **
    (b) CONNECT for Health Act
    (c) Affordable Care Act
    (d) Century Cures Act
2. What individuals are most appropriate for home healthcare services?
    (a) Those with low IQs
    (b) Those with mobility limitations
    (c) Those with severe medical conditions
    (d) **B and C****
3. Which of the following is a benefit of home healthcare services?
    (a) Reduced exposure to infectious diseases
    (b) Provision of informal medical care
    (c) Significant cost savings to the Medicare Program
    (d) **A and C****
4. Which of the following is not considered a home healthcare service?
    (a) **Companion care****
    (b) Occupational Therapy
    (c) Skilled Nursing
    (d) Physical Therapy
5. What is the fundamental purpose of this book?
    (a) To identify providers who play significant roles in the provision of home healthcare services for older patients
    (b) To promote understanding of the care needs of older patients
    (c) **To foster collaborative relationships amongst home healthcare providers who provide care to older patients in the home setting** **
    (d) To provide definitions of interprofessional collaboration

Chapter 2

Discussion Questions

1. Define professionalism and explain its importance throughout the provision of home care services for older adults.

Professionalism is the conduct, aims, or qualities that characterize or mark a profession or a professional. It consists of one's professional parameters, behaviours, and responsibilities. Professionalism is key in ensuring clients receive adequate and acceptable care within the delicate setting of the home without the older individual's loss of dignity, autonomy, or confidentiality. This is why it is vital to emphasize the importance of professionalism, as well as the correlation between this concept and the provision of quality home care services provided to the older adult.

Varied Response

2. What are some of the shared professional dispositions amongst the interprofessional team discussed in this chapter for healthcare personnel in the provision of home care services?
   Some shared professional dispositions for healthcare personnel in the provision of home care services include the commitment to competence, commitment to conduct, and commitment to onfidentiality.

   Varied Response

3. Why is good clinical documentation necessary in healthcare?
   It is the source for patient information, necessary for interprofessional communication, reimbursement for services, and risk management.

   Varied Response

4. Discuss three models that can be used to facilitate cross-cultural communication in healthcare for older adults.
   (a) L.E.A.R.N. Model – Skills for Clinical Care
   (b) R.E.S.P.E.C.T. Model – Building Cross-Cultural Trust
   (c) Iceberg Model – when interacting with older adults, it is necessary to consider the visible (conscious aspects) and unseen (unconscious aspects) of communication.

   Varied Response

Multiple Choice Questions

1. Which of the following are three aspects of professional conduct as discussed in this chapter?

   (a) Respect for the client
   (b) Respect for the profession
   (c) Respect for the professional relationship
   (d) **All of the following****

2. All members of the interprofessional team who provide home care services to older adults are expected to abide by certain ethical expectations and standards as dictated by their individual profession.

   (a) **True****
   (b) False

3. The Healthcare Insurance Portability and Accountability Act of 1996 is a federal law that safeguards the privacy and security of patient information except for which of the following?

   (a) Medical diagnosis or condition
   (b) Treatment services and progress
   (c) **Employment records****
   (d) Demographic Information

4. In clinical documentation, what is the MOST important characteristic of a patient goal? The goal is…

   (a) Concise
   (b) **Functional****
   (c) Flexible
   (d) Idealistic

5. A therapist meets with the wife of a 70-year-old man. The wife informs the therapist that her husband is receiving home health services following a total hip replacement. The client is concerned that her husband is not receiving adequate care because he appears weaker and fearful. She shares that he has developed bed sores and is becoming increasingly withdrawn. The client would like to change to another home care agency. How should the therapist proceed?

   (a) Honour the client's self-determination and assist her in identifying in-home care.
   (b) Assess further for potential elder abuse to determine if a report is required.
   (c) **Inform the client a report is mandated and provide verbal and written report to both law enforcement and the local ombudsman. ****
   (d) Consult with colleagues to determine if this information rises to the level of reasonable suspicion of abuse.

Chapter 3

Discussion Question

1. When considering the case of Jeralean, in what areas could she and her family be assisted with health literacy services and how might that service positively and/or negatively impact them?

   Varied Response

Multiple Choice Questions

1. Which of the following best describes the term patient-centeredness?

   (a) **The interprofessional team approach to healthcare that places the patient at the centre of care delivery and ensures that the patient's needs and values drive the guide clinical decisions. ****
   (b) The interprofessional healthcare team meets with the patient and the caregiver in the patient's home to instruct the caregiver on techniques to provide quality care and assess the caregiver's ability to care for the patient.
   (c) The team of healthcare providers meets with patients and families in a home environment to ensure that the caregiver is providing quality care to the patient.
   (d) Interprofessional healthcare teams work collaboratively to decide what is best for the patient, based on their knowledge, expertise, and clinical judgment.

2. In 2010, the World Health Organization released a Framework for Interprofessional Education and Collaborative Practice. Which of the following statements is TRUE about the WHO Framework for IPECP?

   (a) The framework provides guidelines for healthcare professionals to learn from one another in academic settings.
   (b) The framework provides guidelines for healthcare professionals to work collaboratively in clinical practice settings to develop and implement healthcare plans as a team.
   (c) The framework promotes teams that are founded on mutual respect, shared values, and positive communication.
   (d) **All of these statements are true regarding the WHO framework for interprofessional education and collaborative practices. ****

3. Health literacy is BEST defined as:

   (a) **The degree to which individuals have the ability to find, understand, and use information and services to inform health-related decisions and actions for themselves and others. ****
   (b) A patient who has achieved the highest level of difficulty in reading and understanding medical information related to his or her health condition.
   (c) The capacity of a patient to determine the best course of care for themselves or their family members based on their reading comprehension.
   (d) The ability of the person to gather health information from the Internet and social media sources to learn about health conditions.

4. Which of the following BEST defines caregiver burden?

   (a) **Caregiver burden is best defined as the strain or load of the person who is responsible for caring for a chronically ill, disabled, or older person**

that can impact the well-being and quality of life of both the patient and the caregiver. **

(b) Caregiver burden is best defined as the cross the caregiver must bear for the blessing they have received in life or the blessing they hope to receive in the future.

(c) Caregiver burden refers to the cost of providing quality healthcare in the home environment related to the modifications and adaptations that the caregiver is required to make.

(d) Caregiver burden refers to the physical lifting required by caregivers to assist patients who can't move from one surface to another or transition into different positions.

5. What is the primary role of the caregiver on the interprofessional healthcare team?

   (a) **The primary role of the caregiver is to provide continuous support in a healing relationship for the patient whenever and wherever it is needed. ****

   (b) The primary role of the caregiver is to follow the instructions of the healthcare professionals and communicate them to the patient.

   (c) The primary role of the caregiver is to ensure that the healthcare providers show respect for the patient, keep their scheduled appointments, and report to the physician or home health agency about the quality of each healthcare provider.

   (d) All of the above

6. Who are the caregivers?

   (a) **Caregivers tend to be spouses, partners, family members, or neighbours who often assume the role without much training and preparation. ****

   (b) Caregivers are individuals from a home health agency whose sole purpose is to assist with daily activities and chores.

   (c) Caregivers are typically the men of the family who can provide the most financial support for the patient.

   (d) Caregivers are the individuals and family members who volunteer to care for patients because they have the most time and energy to support the patient.

Chapter 4

Discussion Questions

1. Describe the risk and benefits of providing home care services to older clients and patients?

   Varied Response

2. Why is it important that families have an emergency preparedness plan?

   Varied Response

Assignment

Imagine Jeralean residing in your community. Search the Internet and locate at least five available home care facilities to assist Jeralean in staying in her home. Also, explain how these facilities are similar or different from each other.

Assignment: "Make a Plan" Activity

1. Medical social workers are critical in assisting seniors and their caregivers in the disaster preparedness and response plan. Use the provided emergency preparedness checklist to create your emergency plan.

   Completing this "make a plan" activity will help you know what to do in an emergency. It will take you about 20 minutes to make your plan. Your family may not be together when an emergency happens. Plan on how to meet or contact one another and discuss what you would do in different situations. Finally, keep this document on an easy-to-find emergency kit in case of an emergency.
2. Visit the local Council on Aging or Area resources on elder abuse prevention. What are some of the resources or information you found?

Chapter 5

Discussion Question

1. What is the role of the skilled nurse on the interprofessional team?

   Varied Response

Multiple-Choice Questions

1. What are the priorities that should be established when assessing a patient's home during the initial visit?

   (a) Determine the pharmacy of choice.
   (b) Ask the physician what they want should be done.
   (c) **Assess physical environment; establish patient care needs and expectations.*****
   (d) Determine how best to conduct the home visit.

2. You are visiting your patient in the home setting for the third visit, and the patient tells you "my legs just keep getting weaker, the older I get." Which of the following would be the best action to take?

   (a) **Consult with your team leader for a Physical Therapy Assessment.****
   (b) Ask the patient to walk throughout the house for an assessment.

(c) Tell the patient, "no worries, this is expected as you get older".
(d) Continue with your assessment and care.

3. Which of the following clinicians are not considered interprofessional team members? Select all that apply.

(a) The Provider (MD, APRN, PA)
(b) The Nurse
(c) The Social Worker
(d) The Home Health Aide
(e) **The Patient****

4. When describing skilled nursing care, which of the following is not considered to be an essential component?

(a) **Services from licensed nurses at the hospital****
(b) Services from licensed nurses at home or in a nursing home
(c) Care Services from therapists or technicians in the home
(d) Care Services from aids or other assistive personnel in the home or facility

5. Which of the following is an advantage of the home care (natural) setting?

(a) Persons living in home may create barriers to care.
(b) Potential for lack of sleep, rest periods due to personal and or/family responsibilities or activities.
(c) Potential safety risks for care providers.
(d) **Patient can feel more at ease in natural setting.****

Chapter 6

Discussion Question

Considering the APTA guide to physical therapy practice, when on an interprofessional team providing physical therapy services to an older patient, during which step(s) would interprofessional communication take place and what information would be shared relevant to the step(s) identified.

Varied Response

Multiple Choice Questions

1. Which of the following statements is ***true*** about Physical Therapists?

(a) Physical Therapists are considered movement experts.
(b) PTs help patients to regain the functional independence necessary to maintain their quality of life.

(c) PT interventions can help to reduce the impact, severity, and duration of an illness or injury.
(d) **All of these statements are true. ****

2. Physical therapists treat patients with physical therapist assistants. Which of the following statements is ***false*** about PTAs?

(a) PTAs are licensed by the State Board of Physical Therapy in the jurisdiction in which they practice.
(b) PTAs must graduate from an accredited institution of higher education with a PTA program.
(c) Physical Therapist Assistants must be supervised by a licensed Physical Therapist.
(d) **Physical Therapist Assistants are trained on the job by physicians, PTs, or nurses. ****

3. Physical Therapists use a framework for patient care called the ***patient client management model.*** The ***Patient Client Management Model*** includes which of the following components?

(a) **Examination, evaluation, diagnosis, prognosis and plan of care, interventions, and outcomes****
(b) Plan of care, home assessments, performance-based measures, and interventions for safety
(c) Therapeutic Exercises, Fall Prevention, Patient Education
(d) Interventions, outcomes, diagnosis, and prognosis

4. Which of the following statements is ***true*** regarding older patients?

(a) Older patients are more likely to live with their children after 65 years of age.
(b) **The majority of older patients aged 50 and older want to remain in their homes and communities as they age. ****
(c) Older patients have difficulty adhering to home health appointments.
(d) Older patients tend to prefer to go to outpatient clinics for physical therapy.

5. In order to reduce fall risks, the physical therapist works with the patient and caregiver, and the interprofessional team to ensure that the home environment is safe. Which of the following is considered a safety hazard in home healthcare?

(a) Lifting and moving patients
(b) Clutter and throw rugs on the floors
(c) Pets and hostile animals on the property
(d) **All of these are considered safety hazards****

Chapter 7

Discussion Questions

1. What is the occupational therapist's role in the provision of home care services?
   The profession of occupational therapy is founded on the therapeutic use of occupations and use of self to achieve purposeful and meaningful patient outcomes. The occupational therapist's role of using occupations as a therapeutic tool, as well as client outcomes are ideal to accentuate the provision of home care service for older adults.
2. How does the occupational therapist use the home environment in accentuating the assessment of a client's needs?
   Home environments increase the opportunities to locate available supports and barriers within the home are also able to be easily identified in comparison to office settings. Within the natural settings of clients, the occupational therapist can set treatment plans based upon the person's daily habits and routines with their natural tools and setup.
3. Discuss how the profession of occupational therapy supports the integration of interprofessional partnerships.
   The integration of occupational therapy services into an interprofessional collaborative team is well supported by the American Occupational Therapy Association (AOTA) and that AOTA affirms that occupational therapy practitioners are trained to be direct care providers, consultants, educators, case managers, and advocates for clients and their families. In addition, the AOTA's Vision 2025, supports occupational therapy services interprofessional partnership between occupational therapy and "all people" to be necessary to "maximize health, well-being, and quality of life".

Multiple Choice Questions

1. Natural environments are more disruptive for clients than the office location because they are built into the client's daily routines and are supportive for the client and his or her families as they participate in everyday activities.
   (a) True
   (b) **False****
2. Which of the following supports occupational therapy services interprofessional partnership between occupational therapy and "all people" to be necessary to "maximize health, well-being, and quality of life"? Choose the best answer.
   (a) AOTA's Code of Ethics
   (b) **AOTA's Vision 2025****
   (c) AOTA's Mission
   (d) None of the above

3. The following public health tool is often defined as the use of communications technologies to provide healthcare from a distance.

   (a) Teleporting
   (b) Telephone Communications
   (c) **Telehealth****
   (d) Telegram

4. Older adults need to consider the environmental factors of their homes, including environmental obstacles and design factors. All of the following are safety considerations that may assist older adults in their home environment except which? Please choose the best answer.

   (a) Adding colour contrast
   (b) Increasing lighting
   (c) Removing clutter
   (d) **Adding decorative rugs****

5. Which of the following healthcare professions emphasize the therapeutic use of everyday life occupations for the intent of improving or supporting participation and engagement in one's daily occupation?

   (a) Speech Therapy
   (b) **Occupational Therapy****
   (c) Physical Therapy
   (d) Behavioural Therapy

Chapter 8

Discussion Questions

1. What are common causes of mental illness or psychological distress in older adults?
   Varied Response
2. Give a specific example of an opportunity for a behavioural health professional to collaborate with an interprofessional team member.
   Varied Response

Multiple Choice Questions

1. Behavioural health emphasizes the importance of mental health but also promotes:

   (a) Financial literacy and stability
   (b) Coping and adjustment
   (c) **Health and wellness****

(d) Community engagement

2. Examples of behavioural health professionals include:

   (a) Nutritionists
   (b) Geriatric Counsellors
   (c) Psychiatrists
   (d) **B and C****

3. In primary care settings, behavioural health screenings are typically conducted:

   (a) Over the telephone when the initial appointment is made
   (b) During the initial appointment paperwork
   (c) At the conclusion of the medical appointment
   (d) **Prior to contact with physicians, physician assistants, or nurse practitioners****

4. Which of the following are appropriate behavioural health activities to use with older clients?

   (a) Activities focusing on estate planning
   (b) Activities focusing on memory loss
   (c) Activities focusing on grief and loss
   (d) **B and C****

5. Which of the following is a scale most commonly used to diagnose anxiety?

   (a) **Panic Frequently Questionnaire****
   (b) Mini Mental Status Exam
   (c) Lawton Instrumental Activities of Daily Living Scale
   (d) Beck Depression Inventory

Chapter 9

Discussion Question

1. Consider the following: Your patient demonstrates the ability to don and doff the device properly; however, when therapy arrives, you notice the patient constantly has their prosthesis removed. What are some recommendations that could be provided to the patient to ensure compliance?
   Varied Response

Multiple Choice Questions

1. Which of the following dietary conditions may NOT require referral to a registered dietician?

(a) **Tonsillitis** **
(b) Ill-fitting dentures
(c) Chronic alcohol use
(d) Depression

2. Micronutrient deficiencies can be physically observed in which of the body's structures?

(a) Hair
(b) Muscular System
(c) Skeletal System
(d) **All of the above** **

3. Examples of durable medical equipment include all but which of the following?

(a) Blood glucose meters
(b) Wheelchairs
(c) Dialysis Machine
(d) **Shower Chair** **

4. Which of the following is a primary concern for prosthetic patients?

(a) Sweat management
(b) Sock management
(c) **Pain management** **
(d) Range of motion

5. Which of the following may present a challenge for the orthotist in the home setting?

(a) Over-protective family members
(b) **Working with minimal tools****
(c) The presence of small children in the home
(d) Poor air quality in the home

6. What care model do prosthetists and orthotists adhere to?
(a) National Care Model (NCM)
(b) Prosthetic and Orthotic Quality Care Framework (POQCF)
(c) **International Classification of Functioning, Disability, and Health (ICF)****
(d) None of the above

Assignment to apply to the main case study in Chap. 2:

Consider Jeralean; summarize the findings and potential considerations that the healthcare team must consider when working with this patient. Think back to the home environment and potential obstacles that the patient might encounter. What other factors or considerations would you advise the patient on, for example, referral for other health conditions or considerations?

Chapter 10

Discussion Question

Compare and contrast the 3 definitions of "Quality of Care":

Hoyle (2009) defined quality of care as the "degree to which a set of inherent characteristics fulfils requirements" (p. 24). The Institute of Medicine (National Academy of Medicine) rendered the following definition: "...the degree to which health services for individuals and populations increase the likelihood of desired health outcomes and are consistent with current professional knowledge" (p. 1990, p. 21), and further outlined the six domains of quality of care: safety; effectiveness; patient-centeredness; timeliness; efficiency; and equity (2001, pp. 39–40). The authors of this book have adopted their own definition of quality of care:

The term "quality of care" is best defined as a conceptual model that drives: (a) care planning; (b) patient engagement, progress, and satisfaction; and (c) the conscientious work of interprofessional team members. The term conscientious describes a team member who is reliable, punctual, accountable, ethical; discerning of patient needs/strengths and patient risk/protective factor; and committed to adhering to policies and procedures.

Varied Response

Multiple Choice Questions

1. All home care interventions must be planned, implemented, and monitored with the best interest of ____________ in mind.
   (a) the family
   (b) **the patient****
   (c) the interprofessional team
   (d) the patient and family
2. What is the primary objective of this book?
   (a) To increase the reader's knowledge of various healthcare disciplines
   (b) To increase the reader's knowledge of the health needs of older patients
   (c) **To increase the reader's knowledge of the health needs of older patients from an interprofessional collaborative perspective****
   (d) To increase the reader's knowledge of quality and best practices within the home care setting
3. Which of the following principles of care should continue throughout the episode of care, from the initial visit until care termination?
   (a) Informed consent
   (b) Quality assurance activities

   (c) Timely and accurate documentation and reporting
   (d) **All of the above****

4. Which of the following is an example of asynchronous communication?

   (a) **Communication via a healthcare portal****
   (b) Zoom meeting
   (c) Phone conference
   (d) In-person meeting

5. Ideally, a service quality check should be conducted:

   (a) **During each home visit****
   (b) At least monthly
   (c) At least quarterly
   (d) During discharge

Appendix B: Resource List

1. The National Organization on Disabilities Emergency Preparedness Initiative:
   https://www.nod.org/mission/
2. Emergency preparedness.
   http://www.fema.gov/pdf/areyouready/basic_preparedness.pdf
3. Emergency Preparedness for People with Disabilities:
   https://www.ready.gov/disability
4. Emergency Evacuation Preparedness: Taking Responsibility for your safety—A Guide for People with Disabilities and Other Activity Limitations by June, Issacson, Kailes, Disability Policy Consultant
   http://www.jik.com/pubs/EmergencyEvacuation.pdf
5. FEMA-Federal Emergency management agency: Individuals with Special Needs
   https://www.fema.gov/
6. Disability Preparedness Center
   https://disabilitydisasteraccess.org/
7. Centers for Disease Control and Prevention: Emergency Preparedness
   https://emergency.cdc.gov/
8. The Red Cross
   https://www.redcross.org/
9. Food and Drug Administration: State Health Department
   https://www.fda.gov/
10. Central Alabama Aging Consortium
    https://centralalabamaaging.org/
11. Meals on Wheels
    https://www.macoa.org/meals-on-wheels
12. Adult Protective Services
    https://dhr.alabama.gov/adult-protective-services/

13. Home and Community-Based Medicaid Waiver Services
    https://medicaid.alabama.gov/content/6.0_LTC_waivers/6.1_HCBS_Waivers/6.1.2_Elderly_Disabled_Waiver.aspx
14. Alabama Department of Senior Services
    https://alabamaageline.gov/medicaid-waiver-programs/
15. Social Security Administration for information on Medicare and Medicaid
    https://www.ssa.gov/atlanta/southeast/al/alabama.htm

Appendix C: Chapter 6 Assessment Form

Interactive Interprofessional Home Health Assessment Template

Interprofessional Home Health Assessment/Template		
Name:	**Address:**	**Phone No.:**
Date:	**Time In/Out**	**Medical Doctor:**
Medicare/Advantage	**Authorized Visits:**	**WB Status/Precautions:**
Person Completing Assessment		
□ RN □ PT □ SLP/ST □ OT Start of care:	Patient History: Prior Level of Function: Resumption of care Discharge	Caregiver's Name:____________ Home Number:_____________ Family Members 1. 2.
Patient/Caregiver Education: Self-Care Medication Management Home Exercises Gait/Assistive Devise Transfers/Safety	**Historian Completing Form** □Patient □Family Members or other authorized people □The clinician, on behalf of the patient	**Payment Sources** □Medicare □Medicaid □AARP □Blue Cross □United Health Care □Other Commercial Insurance □Other Form of Payment
Vital Signs Blood pressure _____ Heart Rate _____ O2 Sat. _____ Respiratory Rate _____ Speech _____ Hearing _____ Vision _____ Cognition _____	**Assistance Scale:** □0= Independent □1-Requires minimal Assistance or Supervision □2. Requires 50% assistance or supervision □3. Supervision at all times □4. Totally Dependent on another person to perform safety	**Pts tolerance of today's visit** 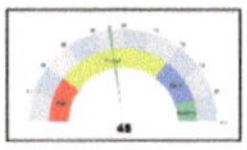 □Red=Poor □Yellow= Fair □Blue=Great □Green=Excellent
Intake	**Body View**	**Review of Systems**
Patient History	Musculoskeletal Status	Sensory Status
Diagnoses	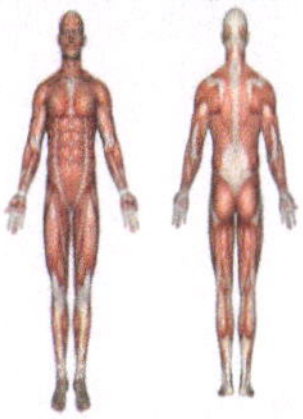	Integumentary Status
Height		Cardiovascular/Pulmonary Status
Weight		Elimination Status
Intake /Output /Elimination		Neuro/Emotional Behavior Status
Living arrangements □Own Home □With Family Members □With Friends □Nursing Home □Others___________ _______________ _______________		**Medical History** Cancer Yes or No Diabetes Yes or No High Blood Pressure Yes or No Heart Disease Yes or No Osteoporosis Yes or No Osteoarthritis Yes or No Prior Surgeries Yes or No Others:______________
	Activities of Daily Living	
Grooming □ Independent □Assisted by Others	**Toilet Transfers** □Independent □Assisted by Others □Bedpan	**Ambulation/Locomotion** □Able to Walk □Crutches/Cane □Assisted by Others □Unable to Determine at this time
Dressing □ Independent □Assisted by Others **Bathing** □ Independent □Assisted by Others	**Toilet Hygiene** □ Independent □ Assisted by Others **Transferring** □Bed □Bedside Commode □Tub	**Feeding/Eating** □ Independent □Assistance Required **Fall Risk Assessment** History of Falls □Yes or □No
Walking	**Mobility**	**Walking**
□Walking 10 feet on uneven surfaces □Walking 15 feet on uneven surfaces □Walker > than 15 feet on uneven surfaces	□Wheelchair or □Scooter □50 feet with two turns □100 feet with four turns	□1 Step curb □ 4 steps □12 steps
Notes:____		eSignature_____________

This versatile tool can be used with smartphones, tablets, and laptops, making it easy for clinicians to store, analyze, and process data for patient care, academic, and research purposes. This tool is a significant advancement, tailored to meet the unique requirements of individual clinicians and support the caregiver and patient in the home environment. The interprofessional assessment allows clinicians to track patients' performance and progress with all team members throughout an episode of care in real time.

This interactive interprofessional assessment form (referenced in Chap. 6 and developed by the authors) enables remote capture and exchange of patient data in real time. This versatile tool can be used with smartphones, tablets, and laptops, making it easy for clinicians to store, analyse, and process data for patient care, academic, and research purposes. This tool is a significant advancement, tailored to meet the unique requirements of individual clinicians and support the caregiver and patient in the home environment. It helps them make informed decisions that promote advocacy, prevention, and the promotion of population health as well as provides up-to-date information to support patients and caregivers[1]. Federal regulations require clinicians to document assessments in the Outcome and Assessment Information Set (OASIS). The interprofessional assessment allows clinicians to track patients' performance and progress with all team members throughout an episode of care in real time.

Reference

1. Kim, S. Y. (2017). Continuity of care. Korean Journal of Family Medicine, *38*(5): 241. doi: 10.4082/kjfm.2017.38.5.241.

Index

D. H. Stapleton, S. Bossie (eds.), *Home Care for Older Adults Using Interprofessional Teams*, https://doi.org/10.1007/978-3-031-40889-2